KETO LUNCH AND SIDE DISHES

KETO LUNCH AND SIDE DISHES

160 Easy To Follow Recipes for Ketogenic
Weight-Loss, Natural Hormonal Health &
Metabolism Boost | Includes a 21 Day Meal Plan

SUZANNE NEWTON

CONTENTS

CONTENTS

CONTENTS

Introduction

Even before we talk about how to do keto – it's important to first consider why this particular diet works. What actually happens to your body to make you lose weight?

As you probably know, the body uses food as an energy source. Everything you eat is turned into energy, so that you can get up and do whatever you need to accomplish for the day. The main energy source is sugar so what happens is that you eat something, the body breaks it down into sugar, and the sugar is processed into energy. Typically, the "sugar" is taken directly from the food you eat so if you eat just the right amount of food, then your body is fueled for the whole day. If you eat too much, then the sugar is stored in your body – hence the accumulation of fat.

But what happens if you eat less food? This is where the Ketogenic Diet comes in. You see, the process of creating sugar from food is usually faster if the food happens to be rich in carbohydrates. Bread, rice, grain, pasta – all of these are carbohydrates and they're the easiest food types to turn into energy.

So the Ketogenic Diet is all about reducing the amount of carbohydrates you eat. Does this mean you won't get the kind of energy you need for the day? Of course not! It only means that now, your body has to find other possible sources of energy. Do you know where they will be getting that energy? Your stored body fat!

So here's the situation – you are eating less carbohydrates every day. To keep you energetic, the body breaks down the stored fat and turns them into molecules called ketone bodies. The process of turning the fat into ketone bodies is called "Ketosis" and obviously – this is where the name of the Ketogenic Diet comes from. The ketone bodies take the place of glucose in keeping you energetic. As long as you keep your carbohydrates reduced, the body will keep getting its energy from your body fat.

Sounds Simple, Right?

The Ketogenic Diet is often praised for its simplicity and when you look at it properly, the process is really straightforward. The Science behind the effectivity of the diet is also well-documented, and has been proven multiple times by different medical fields. For example, an article on Diet Review by Harvard provided a lengthy discussion on how the Ketogenic Diet works and why it is so effective for those who choose to use this diet.

But Fat Is the Enemy...Or Is It?

No – fat is NOT the enemy. Unfortunately, years of bad science told us that fat is something you have to avoid – but it's actually a very helpful thing for weight loss! Even before we move forward with this book, we'll have to discuss exactly what "healthy fats" are, and why they're actually the good guys. To do this, we need to make a distinction between the different kinds of fat. You've probably heard of them before and it is a little bit confusing at first. We'll try to go through them as simply as possible:

Saturated fat. This is the kind you want to avoid. They're also called "solid fat" because each molecule is packed with hydrogen atoms. Simply put, it's the kind of fat that can easily cause a blockage in your body. It can raise cholesterol levels and lead to heart problems or a stroke. Saturated fat is something you can find in meat, dairy products, and other processed food items. Now, you're probably wondering: isn't the Ketogenic Diet packed with saturated fat? The answer is: not necessarily. You'll find later in the recipes given that the Ketogenic Diet promotes primarily unsaturated fat or healthy fat. While there are definitely many meat recipes in the list, most of these recipes contain healthy fat sources.

Unsaturated Fat. These are the ones dubbed as healthy fat. They're the kind of fat you find in avocado, nuts, and other ingredients you usually find in Keto-friendly recipes. They're known to lower blood cholesterol and actually come in two types: polyunsaturated and monounsaturated. Both are good for your body but the benefits slightly vary, depending on what you're consuming.

Polyunsaturated fat. These are perhaps the best in the list. You know about omega-3 fatty acids right? They're often suggested for people who have heart problems and are recognized as the "healthy" kind of fat. Well, they fall under the category of polyunsaturated fat and are known for reducing risks of heart disease by as much as 19 percent. This is according to a study titled: Effects on coronary heart diseases of increased poly-unsaturated fat in lieu of saturated fat: systematic review & meta-analysis of randomized controlled tests. So where do you get these polyunsaturated fats? You can get them mostly from vegetable and seed oils. These are ingredients you can almost always find in Ketogenic Recipes such as olive oil, coconut oil, and more. If you need more convincing, you should also know that omega-3 fatty acids are actually a kind of polyunsaturated fats and you will find them in deep sea fish like tuna, herring, and salmon.

What Is Keto And Why Is So Important For
Your Health

The health benefits of the Keto diet are not different for men or women, but the speed at which
they are reached does differ. As mentioned, human bodies are a lot different when it comes to the
ways that they are able to burn fats and lose weight. For example, by design women have at least 10%
more body fat than men. No matter how fit you are, this is just an aspect of being a human that you
must consider. Don't be hard on yourself if you notice that it seems like men can lose weight easier that's because they can! What women have in additional body fat, men typically have the same
in muscle mass. This is why men tend to see faster external results, because that added muscle mass

means that their metabolism rates are higher. That increased metabolism means that fat and energy get burned faster. When you are on Keto, though, the internal change is happening right away.

Your metabolism is unique, but it is also going to be slower than a man's by nature. Since muscle is able to burn more calories than fat, the weight just seems to fall off of men, giving them the ability to reach the opportunity for muscle growth quickly. This should not be something that holds you back from starting your Keto journey. As long as you are keeping these realistic bodily factors in mind, you won't be left wondering why it is taking you a little bit longer to start losing weight. This point will come for you, but it will take a little bit more of a process that you must be committed to following through with.

Another unique condition that a woman can experience but a man cannot be PCOS or Polycystic Ovary Syndrome; a hormonal imbalance that causes the development of cysts. These cysts can cause pain, interfere with normal reproductive function, and, in extreme and dangerous cases, burst. PCOS is actually very common among women, affecting up to 10% of the entire female population. Surprisingly, most women are not even aware that they have the condition. Around 70% of women have PCOS that is undiagnosed. This condition can cause a significant hormonal imbalance, therefore affecting your metabolism. It can also inevitably lead to weight gain, making it even harder to see results while following diet plans. In order to stay on top of your health, you must make sure that you are going to the gynecologist regularly.

Menopause is another reality that must be faced by women, especially as we age. Most women begin the process of menopause in their mid-40s. Men do not go through menopause, so they are spared from yet another condition that causes slower metabolism and weight gain. When you start menopause, it is easy to gain weight and lose muscle. Most women, once menopause begins, lose muscle at a much faster rate, and conversely gain weight, despite dieting and exercise regimens. Keto can, therefore, be the right diet plan for you. Regardless of what your body is doing naturally, via processes like menopause, your internal systems are still going to be making the switch from running on carbs to deriving energy from fats.

When the body begins to run on fats successfully, you have an automatic fuel reserving waiting to be burned. It will take some time for your body to do this, but when it does, you will actually be able to eat fewer calories and still feel just as full because your body knows to take energy from the fat that you already have. This will become automatic. It is, however, a process that requires some patience, but being aware of what is actually going on with your body can help you stay motivated while on Keto.

Because a Keto diet reduces the amount of sugar you are consuming, it naturally lowers the amount of insulin in your bloodstream. This can actually have amazing effects on any existing PCOS and fertility issues, as well as menopausal symptoms and conditions like pre-diabetes and Type 2 diabetes. Once your body adjusts to a Keto diet, you are overcoming the things that are naturally in place that can be preventing you from losing weight and getting healthy. Even if you placed your body on a strict diet, if it isn't getting rid of sugars properly, you likely aren't going to see the same results that you will when you try Keto. This is a big reason why Keto can be so beneficial for women.

You might not even realize that your hormones are not in balance until you experience a lifestyle that limits carbs and eliminates sugars. Keto is going to reset this balance for you, keeping your hormones at healthy levels. As a result of this, you will probably find yourself in a better general mood, and with much more energy to get through your days.

For people over 50, there are guidelines to follow when you start your Keto diet. As long as you are following the method properly and listening to what your body truly needs, you should have no more problems than men do while following the plan. What you will have are more obstacles to overcome, but you can do it. Remember that plenty of women successfully follow a Keto diet and see great results. Use these women as inspiration for how you anticipate your own journey to go. On the days when it seems impossible, remember what you have working against you, but more importantly what you have working for you. Your body is designed to go into ketogenesis more than it is designed to store fat by overeating carbs. Use this as a motivation to keep pushing you ahead. Keto is a valid option for you and the results will prove this, especially if you are over the age of 40.

Benefit of Keto Diet

GENERAL KETO BENEFITS

PROVEN WEIGHT LOSS · IMPROVED APPETITE CONTROL · STABLE ENERGY · LOWER BLOOD SUGAR LEVELS · LOWER INSULIN LEVELS

ENHANCED FAT BURNING · ENHANCED COGNITIVE PERFORMANCE · CLEANER ENERGY PRODUCTION · DECREASED SYSTEMIC INFLAMMATION · THERAPEUTIC POTENTIAL FOR CERTAIN CANCERS · GLYCOGEN ENHANCEMENT

Benefits Ketogenic Diet

Reduction of cravings and appetite

Many people gain weight simply because they cannot control their cravings and appetite for caloric foods. The ketogenic diet helps eliminate these problems, but it does not mean that you will never be hungry or want to eat. You will feel hungry but only when you have to eat. Several studies have shown that the less carbohydrates you eat, the less you eat overall. Eating healthier foods that are high in fat helps reduce your appetite, as you lose more weight faster on a low-fat diet. The reason for this is that low carbohydrate diets help lower insulin levels, as your body does not need too much insulin to convert glycogen to glucose while eliminating excess water in your body. This diet helps you reduce visceral fat. In this way, you will get a slimmer look and shape. It is the most difficult fat to lose, as it surrounds the organs as it increases. High doses can cause inflammation and insulin resistance. Coconut oil can produce an immediate source of energy as it increases ketone levels in your body.

Reduction of risk of heart disease

Triglycerides, fat molecules in your body, have close links with heart disease. They are directly proportional as the more the number of triglycerides, the higher your chances of suffering from heart disease. You can reduce the number of free triglycerides in your body by reducing the number of carbohydrates, as is in the keto diets.

Reduces chances of having high blood pressure

Weight loss and blood pressure have a close connection; thus, since you are losing weight while on the keto diet, it will affect your blood pressure.

Fights type 2 diabetes

Type two diabetes develops as a result of insulin resistance. This is a result of having huge amounts of glucose in your system, with the keto diet this is not a possibility due to the low carbohydrate intake.

Increases the production of HDL

High-density lipoprotein is referred to as good cholesterol. It is responsible for caring calories to your liver, thus can be reused. High fat and low carbohydrate diets increase the production of HDL in your body, which also reduces your chances of getting a heart disease. Low-density lipoprotein is referred to as bad cholesterol.

Suppresses your appetite

It is a strange but true effect of the keto diet. It was thought that this was a result of the production of ketones but this was proven wrong as a study taken between people on a regular balanced diet and some on the keto diet and their appetites were generally the same. It, however, helps to suppress appetite as it is it has a higher fat content than many other diets. Food stays in the stomach for longer as fat and is digested slowly, thus provides a sense of fullness. On top of that, proteins promote the secretion cholecystokinin, which is a hormone that aids in regulating appetite. It is also believed that the ketogenic diet helps to suppress your appetite by continuous blunting of appetite. There is increased appetite in the initial stages of the diet, which decreases over time.

Changes in cholesterol levels

This is kind of on the fence between good and bad. This is because the ketogenic diet involves a high fat intake which makes people wonder about the effect on blood lipids and its potential to increase chances of heart disease and strokes, among others. Several major components play a lead role in determining this, which is: LDL, HDL, and blood triglyceride levels. Heart disease correlates with high levels of LDL and cholesterol. On the other hand, high levels of HDL are seen as protection from diseases caused by cholesterol levels. The impacts of the diet on cholesterol are not properly known. Some research has shown that there is no change in cholesterol levels while others have said that there is change. If you stay in deep ketosis for a very long period of time, your blood lipids will increase, but you will have to go through some negative effects of the ketogenic diet which will be corrected when the diet is over. If a person does not remain following the diet strictly for like ten years, he/she will not experience any cholesterol problems. It is difficult to differentiate the difference between diet and weight loss in general. The effect of the ketogenic diet on cholesterol has been boiled down to if you lose fat on the ketogenic diet then your cholesterol levels will go down, and if you don't lose fat, then your cholesterol levels will go up. Strangely, women have a larger cholesterol level addition than men, while both are on a diet. As there is no absolute conclusion on the effect of the ketogenic diet on cholesterol, you are advised to have your blood lipid levels constantly checked for any bad effects. Blood lipid levels should be checked before starting the diet and about eight weeks after starting. If repeated results show a worsening of lipid levels, then you should abandon the diet or substitute saturated fats with unsaturated fats.

Risk of a Ketogenic Diet

Low energy levels

When available, the body prefers to use carbohydrates for fuel as they burn more effectively than fats. General drop-in energy level is a concern raised by many dieters due to the lack of carbohydrates. Studies have shown that it causes orthostatic hypotension which causes lightheadedness. It has come to be known that these effects can be avoided by providing enough supplemental nutrients like sodium. Many of the symptoms can be prevented by providing 5 grams of sodium per day. Most times, fatigue disappears after a few weeks or even days, if fatigue doesn't disappear, then you should add a small number of carbohydrates to the diet as long as ketosis is maintained. The diet is not recommended when caring out high-intensity workouts, weight training, or high-intensity aerobic exercise as carbohydrates are an absolute requirement but are okay for low-intensity exercise.

Effects on the brain

It causes increased use of ketones by the brain. The increased use of ketones, among other reasons, result in the treating of childhood epilepsy. As a result of the changes that occur, the concern over the side effects, including permanent brain damage and short-term memory loss, has been raised. The origin of these concerns is difficult to understand. The brain is powered by ketones in the absence of glucose. Ketones are normal energy sources and not toxic as the brain creates enzymes, during fetal growth, that helps us use them. Epileptic children, though not the perfect examples, show some insight into the effects of the diet on the brain in the long term. There is no negative effect in terms of cognitive function. There is no assurance that the diet cannot have long term dietary effects, but no information proves that there are any negative effects. Some people feel they can concentrate more when on the ketogenic diet, while others feel nothing but fatigue. This is as a result of differences in individual physiology. There are very few studies that vaguely address the point on short term memory loss. This wore off with the continuation of the study.

Kidney stones and kidney damage

As a result of the increased workload from having to filter ketones, urea, and ammonia, as well as dehydration concerns of the potential for kidney damage or passing kidney stones have been raised. The high protein nature of the ketogenic diet raises the alarms of individuals who are concerned with potential kidney damage. There is very little information that points to any negative effects of the diet on kidney function or development of kidney stones. There is a low incidence of small kidney stones in epileptic children this may be as a result of the state of deliberate dehydration that the children are put at instead of the ketosis state itself. Some short term research shows no change in kidney function or increased incidents of kidney stones either after they are off the diet or after six months on a diet. There is no long term data on the effects of ketosis to kidney function; thus, no complete conclusions can be made. People with preexisting kidney issues are the only ones who get problems from high protein intake. From an unscientific point of view, one would expect increased incidents of this to happen to athletes who consume very high protein diets, but it has not happened. This suggests that high protein intake, under normal conditions, is not harmful to the kidneys. To limit the possibility of kidney stones, it is advised to drink a lot of water to maintain hydration. For people who are predisposed to kidney stones should have their kidney function should be monitored to ensure that no complications arise if they decide to follow through with the diet.

Constipation

A common side effect of the diet is reduced bowel movements and constipation. This arises from two different causes: lack of fiber and gastrointestinal absorption of foods. First, the lack of carbs in the diet means that unless supplements are taken, fiber intake is low. Fiber is very important to our systems. High fiber intake can prevent some health conditions, including heart disease and some forms of cancer. Use some type of sugar-free fiber supplement to prevent any health problems and help you maintain regular bowel movements. The diet also reduces the volume of stool due to enhanced absorption and digestion of food; thus, fewer waste products are generated.

Fat regain

Dieting, in general, has very low long term success rates. There are some effects of getting out of a ketogenic diet like the regain of fat lost through calorific restriction alone. This is true for any diet based on calorific restriction. It is expected for weight to be regained after carb reintroduction. For people who use the weighing scale to measure their success, they may completely shun carbs as they think it is the main reason for the weight regain. You should understand that most of the initial weight gain is water and glycogen.

Immune system

There is a large variety in the immunity system response to ketogenic diets on different people. There has been some repost on reduction on some ailments such allergies and increased minor sickness susceptibility.

Optic neuropathy

This is optic nerve dysfunction. It has appeared in a few cases, but it is still existence. It was linked to the people not getting adequate amounts of calcium or vitamins supplements for about a year. All the cases were corrected by supplementation of adequate vitamin B, especially thiamine.

Some Tips for Beginner to Achieve Keto Success

Nobody told you that life was going to be this way! But don't worry. There's still plenty of time to make amendments and take care of your health. Here are a couple of tips that will allow you to lead a healthier life in your fifties:

Start Building on Immunity

Every day, our body is exposed to free radicals and toxins from the environment. The added stress of work and family problems doesn't make it any easier for us. To combat this, it's essential that you start consuming healthy veggies that contain plenty of antioxidants and build a healthier immune system.

This helps ward off unwanted illnesses and diseases, allowing you to maintain good health.

Adding more healthy veggies to your Keto diet will help you obtain a variety of minerals, vitamins and antioxidants.

Consider Quitting Smoking

It's never too late to try to quit smoking even if you are in your fifties. Once a smoker begins to quit, the body quickly starts to heal the previous damages caused by smoking.

Once you start quitting, you'll notice how you'll be able to breathe easier, while acquiring a better sense of smell and taste. Over the period of time, eliminating the habit of smoking can greatly reduce the risks of high blood pressure, strokes and heart attack. Please note how these diseases are much more common among folks who are in the fifties and above when compared to younger folks.

Not to mention, quitting smoking will help you stay more active and enjoy better health with your friends and family.

Stay Social

We've already mentioned this before but it's worth pondering on again and again. Aging can be a daunting process and trying to get through it all on your own isn't particularly helpful. We urge you to stay in touch with friends and family or become a part of a local community club or network. Some older folks find it comforting to get an emotional support animal.

Being surrounded by people you love will give you a sense of belonging and will improve your mood. It'll also keep your mind and memory sharp as you engage in different conversations.

Health Screenings You Should Get After Your Fifties

Your fifties are considered the prime years of your life. Don't let the joy of these years be robbed away from you because of poor health. Getting simple tests done can go a long way in identifying any potential health problems that you may have. Here is a list of health screenings should get done:

Check Your Blood Pressure

Your blood pressure is a reliable indicator of your heart health. In simple words, blood pressure is a measure of how fast blood travels through the artery walls. Very high or even very low blood pressure can be a sign of an underlying problem. Once you hit your 40s, you should have your blood pressure checked more often.

EKG

The EKG reveals your heart health and activity. Short for electrocardiogram, the EKG helps identify problems in the heart. The process works by highlighting any rhythm problems that may be in the heart such as poor heart muscles, improper blood flow or any form of abnormality. Getting an EKG is also a predictive measure for understanding the chances of a heart attack. Since people starting their fifties are at greater risk of getting a heart attack, you should get yourself checked more often.

Mammogram

Mammograms help rule out the risks of breast cancer. Women who enter their fifties should ideally get a mammogram after every ten years. However, if you have a family history, it is advisable that you get one much earlier to rule out the possibilities of cancer.

Blood Sugar Levels

If you're somebody who used to grab a fast food meal every once in a while before you switched to Keto, then you should definitely check your blood sugar levels more carefully. Blood sugar levels indicate whether or not you have diabetes. And you know how the saying goes, prevention is better than cure. It's best to clear these possibilities out of the way sooner than later.

Check for Osteoporosis

Unfortunately, as you grow older you also become susceptible to a number of bone diseases. Osteoporosis is a bone-related condition in which bones begin to lose mass, becoming frail and weak. Owing to this, seniors become more prone to fractures. This can make even the smallest of falls detrimental to your health.

Annual Physical Exam

Your insurance must be providing coverage for your annual physical exam. So, there's no reason you should not take advantage of it. This checkup helps identify the state of your health. You'll probably be surprised by how much doctors can tell from a single blood test.

Prostrate Screening Exam

Once men hit their fifties, they should be screened for prostate cancer (similar to how women should get a mammogram and pap smear). Getting a screening done becomes especially important if cancer runs in your family.

Eye Exam

As you start to age, you'll notice how your eyesight will start to deteriorate. It's quite likely that vision is not as sharp as it used to be. Ideally, you should have gotten your first eye exam during your 40s but it isn't too late. Get one as soon as possible to prevent symptoms from escalating.

Be Wary of Any Weird Moles

While skin cancer can become a problem at any age, older adults should pay closer attention to any moles or unusual skin tags in their bodies. While most cancers can be easily treated, melanoma can be particularly quite dangerous. If you have noticed any recent moles in your body that have changed in color, size or shape, make sure to visit the dermatologist.

Check Your Cholesterol Levels

Now, we've talked about this plenty of times but it's worth mentioning again. High cholesterol levels can be dangerous to your health and can be an indicator for a number of diseases, things become more complicated for conditions that don't show particular symptoms. Just to be on the safe side, your total cholesterol levels should be below 200 mg per deciliter. Your doctor will take a simple blood test and will give you a couple of guidelines with the results. In case there is something to worry about, you should make serious dietary and lifestyle changes in your life.

What does the ketogenic diet mean to women?

Women who are looking for a quick and effective way to shed excess weight, get high blood sugar levels under control, reduce overall inflammations, and improve physical and mental energy will do their best by following a ketogenic diet plan. But there are special considerations women must take into account when they are beginning the keto diet.

All women know it is much more difficult for women to lose weight than it is for men to lose weight. A woman will live on a starvation level diet and exercise like a triathlete and only lose five pounds. A man will stop putting dressing on his salad and will lose twenty pounds. It just is not fair.

But we have the fact that we are women to blame. Women naturally have more standing between them and weight loss than men do.

The mere fact that we are women is the largest single contributor to the reason we find it difficult to lose weight. Since our bodies always think they need to be prepared for the possibility of pregnancy women will naturally have more body fat and less mass in our muscles than men will. Muscle cells burn more calories than fat cells do. So, because we are women, we will always lose weight more slowly than men will.

Being in menopause will also cause women to add more pounds to their bodies, especially in the lower half of the body. After menopause a woman's metabolism naturally slows down. Your hormones levels will decrease. These two factors alone will cause weight gain in the post-menopausal woman.

Women are a direct product of their hormones. Men also have hormones but not the ones like we have that regulate every function in our bodies. And the hormones in women will fluctuate around their everyday habits like lack of sleep, poor eating habits, and menstrual cycles. These hormones cause women to crave sweets around the time their periods occur. These cravings will wreck any diet plan. Staying true to the keto plan is challenging at this time because of the intense craving for sweets and carbs. Also having your period will often make you feel and look bloated because of the water your body holds onto during this time. And having cramps make you more likely to reach for a bag of cookies than a plate of steak and salad.

Because we are women, we may experience challenges on the keto diet that men will not face because they are men. One of these challenges is having weight loss plateau or even experiencing weight gain. This can happen because of the influence of hormones on weight loss in women. If this happens you will want to increase your consumption of good fats like ghee, butter, eggs, coconut oil, beef, avocados, and olive oil. Any food that is cooked or prepared using oil must be prepared in olive oil or avocado oil.

You can also use MCT oil. MCT stands for medium chain triglycerides. This is a form of fatty acid that is saturated and has many health benefits. MCT can help with many body functions from weight loss to improved brain function. MCTs are mostly missing from the typical American diet because we have been told that saturated fats are harmful to the body, and as a group they are. But certain saturated fats, like MCTs, are actually beneficial to the body, especially when they come from good foods like beef or coconut oil. They are easier to digest than most other saturated fats and may help improve heart and brain function and prevent obesity.

Many women on a keto diet will struggle with imbalances in their hormones. On the keto diet you do not rely on lowered calories to lose weight but on foods effect on your hormones. So, when women begin the keto diet any issues, they are already having with their hormones will be brought to attention and may cause the woman to give up before she really begins. Always remember that the keto diet is responsible for cleansing the system first so that the body can easily respond to the wonderful affects a keto diet has to offer.

Do not try to work toward the lean body that many men sport. It is best for overall function that women stay at twenty-two to twenty six percent body fat. Our hormones will function best in this range and we can't possibly function without our hormones. Women who are very lean, like gymnasts and extreme athletes, will find their hormones no longer function or function at a less than optimal rate. And remember that ideal weight may not be the right weight for you. Many women find that they perform their best when they are at their happy weight. If you find yourself fighting with yourself to lose the last few pounds you think you need to lose in order to have the perfect body then it may not be worth it. The struggle will affect your hormone function. Carefully observing the keto diet will allow time for your hormones to stabilize and regulate themselves back to their pre-obesity normal function.

Like any other diet plan the keto diet will work better if you are active. Regular exercise will allow the body to strengthen and tone muscles and will help to work off excess fat reserves. But exercise requires energy to accomplish. If you restrict your carb intake too much you might not have the energy needed to be physically able to make it all the way through the day and still be able to maintain an exercise routine. You might need to add in more carbs to your diet through the practice of carb cycling.

As a woman you know that sometimes your emotions get the better of you. This is true with your body, as you well know, and can be a major reason why women find it extremely difficult at times to lose weight the way they want to lose weight. We have been led to believe that not only can we do it all but that we must do it all. This gives many women unnecessary levels of pressure and can cause them to engage in emotional eating. Some women might have lowered feelings of self-worth and may not feel they are entitled to the benefits of the keto diet, and turning to food relieves the feelings of inadequacy that we try to hide from the world.

When you engage in the same activity for a long period of time it becomes a habit. When you reach for the bag of potato chips or the tub of ice cream whenever you are angry, upset, or depressed, then your brain will eventually tell you to reach for food whenever you feel an emotion that you don't want to deal with. Food acts as a security blanket against the world outside. It may be necessary to address any extreme emotional issues you are having before you begin the keto diet, so that you are better assured of success.

The basic act of staying on the keto diet can be very challenging for some women. Many women see beginning a new diet to lose weight as a punishment for being overweight. It may be worthwhile for you to work at changing the set of your mind if you are feeling this way. You may need to remind yourself daily that the keto diet is not a punishment but a blessing for your body. Tell yourself that you are not denying yourself certain foods because you can't eat them, but because you do not like the way those foods make your body feel. Don't watch other people eating their high carb diet and pity yourself. Instead, feel sorry for the people who have trapped themselves in a high calorie diet and are not experiencing the benefits that you are experiencing.

And for the first thirty days cut out all sweeteners, even the non-sugar ones that are allowed on the keto diet. While they may make food taste better, they also remind your brain that it needs sweet foods when it really doesn't. Cutting them out for at least thirty days will break the cycle that your body has fallen into and will cut the cravings for sweets in your diet.

It is very possible for women to be successful on the keto diet if they are prepared to follow a few simple adjustments that will make the diet look differently than your male partner might be eating but that will make you successful in the long run.

During the first one or two weeks you will need to consume extra fat than a man might need to. Doing this will have three important effects on your body. First it will cause your mitochondria to intensify their acceptance of your new way of finding energy. Mitochondria are tiny organisms that are found in cells and are responsible for using the fuel that insulin brings to the cell for fuel for the cell. Increasing your fat intake will also help make sure you are getting enough calories in your daily diet. This is important because if your body thinks you are starving it will begin to conserve calories and you will stop losing weight.

The third benefit from eating more fat, and perhaps the most important, is the psychological boost you will get from seeing that you can eat more fat and still lose weight and feel good. It will also reset your mindset that you formerly might have held against fat. For so long we have been told that low fat is the only way to lose weight. But an absence of dietary fat will lead to overeating and binge eating out of a feeling of deprivation. When you begin the diet by allowing yourself to eat a lot, or too much in your mind, fat, then you swing the pendulum around to the other side of the fat scale where it properly belongs. You teach yourself that fat can be good for you. Increasing the extra intake of fats should not last beyond the second week of the diet. Your body will improve its abilities to create and burn ketones and body fat, and then you will begin using your own body fat for fuel and you can begin to lower your reliance on dietary fat a little bit so that you will begin to lose weight.

The keto diet is naturally lower in calories if you follow the recommended levels of food intake. It is not necessary to try to restrict your intake of calories even further. All you need to do is to eat only until you are full and not one bite more. Besides losing weight the aim of the keto diet is to re-train your body on how to work properly. You will need to learn to trust your body and the signals it sends out to be able to readjust to a proper way of eating.

6

Keto Diet Benefits for Women

TOP 5 KETO DIET BENEFITS FOR WOMEN

ELIMINATE BLOOD SUGAR HIGHS AND LOWS

BALANCE HORMONES FOR BETTER SEX AND FERTILITY

HELP OPTIMIZE BRAIN FUNCTION

GAIN BETTER OVERALL HEALTH FROM INCREASED NUTRIENTS

BECOME BETTER IN TUNE WITH YOUR BODY FOR LIFELONG WELLNESS

Why Keto for Women?

The health benefits of the Keto diet are not different for men or women, but the speed at which they are reached does differ. As mentioned, women's bodies are a lot different when it comes to the ways that they are able to burn fats and lose weight. For example, by design women have at least 10% more body fat than men. No matter how fit you are, this is just an aspect of being a woman that you must consider. Don't be hard on yourself if you notice that it seems like men can lose weight easier — that's because they can! What women have in additional body fat; men typically have the same in muscle mass. This is why men tend to see faster external results, because that added muscle mass means that their metabolism rates are higher. That increased metabolism means that fat and energy get burned faster. When you are on Keto, though, the internal change is happening right away.

Your metabolism is unique, but it is also going to be slower than a man's by nature. Since muscle is able to burn more calories than fat, the weight just seems to fall off of men, giving them the ability to reach the opportunity for muscle growth quickly. This should not be something that holds you back from starting your Keto journey. As long as you are keeping these realistic bodily factors in mind, you won't be left wondering why it is taking you a little bit longer to start losing weight. This point will come for you, but it will take a little bit more of a process that you must be committed to following through with.

Another unique condition that a woman can experience but a man cannot be PCOS or Polycystic Ovary Syndrome; a hormonal imbalance that causes the development of cysts. These cysts can cause pain, interfere with normal reproductive function, and, in extreme and dangerous cases, burst. PCOS is actually very common among women, affecting up to 10% of the entire female population. Surprisingly, most women are not even aware that they have the condition. Around 70% of women have PCOS that is undiagnosed. This condition can cause a significant hormonal imbalance, therefore affecting your metabolism. It can also inevitably lead to weight gain, making it even harder to see results while following diet plans. In order to stay on top of your health, you must make sure that you are going to the gynecologist regularly.

Menopause is another reality that must be faced by women, especially as we age. Most women begin the process of menopause in their mid-40s. Men do not go through menopause, so they are spared from yet another condition that causes slower metabolism and weight gain. When you start menopause, it is easy to gain weight and lose muscle. Most women, once menopause begins, lose muscle at a much faster rate, and conversely gain weight, despite dieting and exercise regimens. Keto can, therefore, be the right diet plan for you. Regardless of what your body is doing naturally, via processes like menopause, your internal systems are still going to be making the switch from running on carbs to deriving energy from fats.

Because a Keto diet reduces the amount of sugar you are consuming, it naturally lowers the amount of insulin in your bloodstream. This can actually have amazing effects on any existing PCOS and fertility issues, as well as menopausal symptoms and conditions like pre-diabetes and Type 2 diabetes. Once your body adjusts to a Keto diet, you are overcoming the things that are naturally in place that can be preventing you from losing weight and getting healthy. Even if you placed your body on a strict diet, if it isn't getting rid of sugars properly, you likely aren't going to see the same results that you will when you try Keto. This is a big reason why Keto can be so beneficial for women.

As we've deliberated, carbs and sugar can have a huge impact on your hormonal balance. You might not even realize that your hormones are not in balance until you experience a lifestyle that limits carbs and eliminates sugars. Keto is going to reset this balance for you, keeping your hormones at healthy levels. As a result of this, you will probably find yourself in a better general mood, and with much more energy to get through your days.

Why Keto for 40+?

As we age, we naturally look for ways to hold onto our youth and energy. It's not uncommon to think about things that promote anti-aging. Products and lifestyle changes are advertised everywhere, and they are designed to catch your attention, as you grapple with the reality of what it means to be a 40+ year-old woman in our society. Even if you aren't eating for the purposes of anti-aging yet, you have likely thought about it in terms of the way you treat your skin and hair, for example. The great thing about the Keto diet is that it supports maximum health, from the inside out; working hard to make sure that you are in the best shape that you can be in.

For instance, indigestion becomes common as you age. This happens because the body is not able to break down certain foods as well as it used to. With all of the additives and fillers, we all become used to putting our bodies through discomfort in an attempt to digest regular meals. You are probably not even aware that you are doing this to your body, but upon trying a Keto diet, you will realize how your digestion will begin to change. You will no longer feel bloated or uncomfortable after you eat. If you notice this as a common feeling, you are likely not eating food that is nutritious enough to satisfy your needs and is only resulting in excess calories.

Keto fills you up in all of the ways that you need, allowing your body to truly digest and metabolize all of the nutrients. When you eat your meals, you should not feel the need to overeat in order to overcompensate for not having enough nutrients. Anything that takes stress off of any system in your body is going to become a form of anti-aging. You will quickly find this benefit once you start your Keto journey, as it is one of the first-reported changes that most participants notice. In addition to a healthier digestive system, you will also experience more regular bathroom usage, with little to none of the problems often associated with age.

While weight loss is one of the more common desires for most 40+ women who start a diet plan, the way that the weight is lost matters. If you have ever shed a lot of weight before, you have probably experienced the adverse effects of sagging or drooping skin that you were left to deal with. Keto actually rejuvenates the elasticity in your skin. This means that you will be able to lose weight and your skin will be able to catch up. Instead of having to do copious amounts of exercise to firm up your skin, it should already be becoming firmer each day that you are on the Keto diet. This is something that a lot of participants are pleasantly surprised to find out.

Women also commonly report a natural reduction in wrinkles, and healthier skin and hair growth, in general. Many women who start the diet report that they actually notice reverse effects in their aging process. While the skin becomes healthier and more supple, it also becomes firmer. Even if you aren't presently losing weight, you will still be able to appreciate the effects that Keto brings to your skin and face. Because your internal systems are becoming healthier by the day, this tends to show on the outside in a short amount of time. You will also begin to feel healthier. While it is possible to read about the experiences of others, there is nothing like feeling this for yourself when you begin Keto.

Everyone, especially women over 40, has day-to-day tasks that are draining and require certain amounts of energy to complete. Aging can, unfortunately, take away from your energy reserve, even if you get enough sleep at night. It limits the way that you have to live your life, and this can become a very frustrating realization. Most diet plans bring about a sluggish feeling that you are simply supposed to get used to, for example. But Keto does the exact opposite. When you change your eating habits to fit the Keto guidelines, you are going to be hit with a boost of energy. Since your body is truly getting everything that it needs nutritionally, it will repay you with a sustained energy supply.

Another common complaint for women over 40 is that, seemingly overnight, your blood sugar levels are going to be more sensitive than usual. While it is important that everyone keeps an eye on these levels, it is especially important for those who are in their 50s and beyond. High blood sugar can be an indication that diabetes is on the way, but Keto can become a preventative measure, that we've already talked about. Additionally, naturally regulating elevated blood sugar levels, also reduces systemic inflammation, which is also common for women over 50. By balancing the immune system, of which inflammation is a part of, common aches and pains are reduced. Inflammation can also affect vital organs and is a precursor to cancer. Keto will support your path to an anti-inflammatory lifestyle.

Sugar is never great for us, but it turns out that sugar can become especially dangerous as we age. What is known as a "sugar sag" can occur when you get older because the excess sugar molecules will attach themselves to skin and protein in your body. This doesn't even necessarily happen because you are eating too much sugar. Average levels of sugar intake can also lead to this sagging as the sugar weakens the strength of your proteins that are supposed to hold you together. With sagging comes even more wrinkles and arterial stiffening.

If you have any anti-aging concerns, the Keto diet will likely be able to address your worries. It is a diet that works extremely hard while allowing you a fairly simple and direct guideline to follow in return. While your motivation is necessary in order to form a successful relationship with Keto, you won't need to worry about doing anything "wrong" or accidentally breaking from your diet. As long as you know how to give up your sugary foods and drinks while making sure that you are consuming the correct amount of carbs, you will be able to find your own success while on the diet.

As a woman over 50, you'll find that you will feel better, healthier and younger, by implementing the simple steps that will tune your body into processing excess fats for energy. You'll build muscle, lose fat, and look and feel younger. As we've touched on, a Keto diet helps balance your hormones, reversing and/or eliminating many common menopausal signs and symptoms.

7

What Keto Does to an over 50 Woman's Body

How the ketogenic diet can aid with the signs and symptoms of ageing and menopause

For ageing women, menopause will bring severe changes and challenges, but the ketogenic diet can help you switch gears effortlessly to continue enjoying a healthy and happy life. Menopause can upset hormonal levels in women, which consequently affects brainpower and cognitive abilities. Furthermore, due to less production of estrogens and progesterone, your sex drive declines, and you suffer from sleep issues and mood problems. Let's have a look at how a ketogenic diet will help solve these side effects.

Enhanced Cognitive Functions

Usually, hormone estrogen ensures continuous flow of glucose into your brain. But after menopause, the estrogen levels begin to drop dramatically, so does the amount of glucose reaching the bran. As a result, your functional brainpower will start to deteriorate. However, by following the keto diet for women over 50, the problem of glucose intake is circumvented. This results in enhanced cognitive functions and brain activity.

Hormonal Balance

Usually, women face major symptoms of menopause due to hormonal imbalances. The keto diet for women over 50 works by stabilizing these imbalances such as estrogen. This aids in experiencing fewer and bearable menopausal symptoms like hot flashes. The keto diet also balances blood sugar levels and insulin and helps in controlling insulin sensitivity.

Intensified Sex Drive

The keto diet surges the absorption of vitamin D, which is essential for enhancing sex drive. Vitamin D ensures stable levels of testosterone and other sex hormones that could become unstable due to low levels of testosterone.

Better Sleep

Glucose disturbs your blood sugar levels dramatically, which in turn leads to poor quality of sleep. Along with other menopausal symptoms, good sleep becomes a huge problem as you age. The keto diet for women over 50 not only balances blood glucose levels, but also stabilizes other hormones like cortisol, melatonin, and serotonin warranting an improved and better sleep.

Reduces inflammation

Menopause can upsurge the inflammation levels by letting potential harmful invaders in our system, which result in uncomfortable and painful symptoms. Keto diet for women over 50 uses the healthy anti-inflammatory fats to reduce inflammation and lower pain in your joints and bones.

Fuel your brain

Are you aware that your brain is composed of 60% fat or more? This infers that it needs a larger amount of fat to keep it functioning optimally. In other words, the ketones from the keto diet serve as the energy source that fuels your brain cells.

Nutrient deficiencies

Ageing women tend to have higher deficiencies in essential nutrients such as, iron deficiency which leads to brain fog and fatigue; Vitamin B12 deficiency, which lead to neurological conditions like dementia; Fats deficiency, that can lead to problems with cognition, skin, vision; and Vitamin D deficiency that not only causes cognitive impairment in older adults and increase the risk of heart disease but also contribute to the risk of developing cancer. On a keto diet, the high-quality proteins ensure adequate and excellent sources of these important nutrients.

Controlling Blood Sugar

Research has suggested a link between poor blood sugar levels and brain diseases such as Alzheimer's disease, Parkinson's disease, or Dementia. Some factors contributing to Alzheimer's disease may include:

- Enormous intake of carbohydrates, especially from fructose—which is drastically reduced in the ketogenic diet.

- Lack of nutritional fats and good cholesterol — which are copious and healthy in the keto diet

Keto diet helps control blood sugar and improve nutrition; which in turn not only improve insulin response and resistance but also protect against memory loss which is often a part of ageing.

8

How Can Ketogenic Diet Can Aid With the Sign and Symptoms of Ageing and Menopause

To make the most of your diet, there are prohibited foods, and others that are allowed, but in limited quantities. Here are the foods allowed in the ketogenic diet:

Food allowed in unlimited quantities

Lean or fatty meats

No matter which meat you choose, it contains no carbohydrates so that you can have fun! Pay attention to the quality of your meat, and the amount of fat. Alternate between fatty meats and lean meats!

Here are some examples of lean meats:

Beef: sirloin steak, roast beef, 5% minced steak, roast, flank steak, tenderloin, Grisons meat, tripe, kidneys

Horse: roti, steak

Pork: tenderloin, bacon, kidneys

Veal: cutlet, shank, tenderloin, sweetbread, liver

Chicken and turkey: cutlet, skinless thigh, ham

Rabbit

Here are some examples of fatty meats:

Lamb: leg, ribs, brain

Beef: minced steak 10, 15, 20%, ribs, rib steak, tongue, marrow

Pork: ribs, brain, dry ham, black pudding, white pudding, bacon, terrine, rillettes, salami, sausage, sausages, and merguez

Veal: roast, paupiette, marrow, brain, tongue, dumplings

Chicken and turkey: thigh with skin

Guinea fowl

Capon

Turkey

Goose: foie gras

Lean or fatty fish

The fish does not contain carbohydrates so that you can consume unlimited! As with meat, there are lean fish and fatty fish, pay attention to the amount of fat you eat and remember to vary your intake of fish. Oily fish have the advantage of containing a lot of good cholesterol, so it is beneficial for protection against cardiovascular disease! It will be advisable to consume fatty fish more than lean fish, to be able to manage your protein intake: if you consume lean fish, you will have a significant protein intake and little lipids, whereas with fatty fish, you will have a balanced protein and fat intake!

Here are some examples of lean fish:

- Cod
- Colin
- Sea bream
- Whiting
- Sole
- Turbot
- Limor career
- Location
- Pike
- Ray

Here are some examples of oily fish:

- Swordfish
- Salmon
- Tuna
- Trout
- Monkfish
- Herring
- Mackerel
- Cod
- Sardine

Eggs

The eggs contain no carbohydrates, so you can consume as much as you want. It is often said that eggs are full of cholesterol and that you have to limit their intake, but the more cholesterol you eat, the less your body will produce by itself! In addition, it's not just poor-quality cholesterol so that you can consume 6 per week without risk! And if you want to eat more but you are afraid for your cholesterol and I have not convinced you, remove the yellow!

Vegetables and raw vegetables

Yes, you can eat vegetables. But you have to be careful which ones: you can eat leafy vegetables (salad, spinach, kale, red cabbage, Chinese cabbage...) and flower vegetables (cauliflower, broccoli, Romanesco cabbage...) as well as avocado, cucumbers, zucchini or leeks, which do not contain many carbohydrates.

The oils

It's oil, so it's only fat, so it's unlimited to eat, but choose your oil wisely! Prefer olive oil, rapeseed, nuts, sunflower or sesame for example!

Foods authorized in moderate quantities.

The cold cuts

As you know, there is bad cholesterol in cold meats, so you will need to moderate your intake: eat it occasionally!

Fresh cheeses and plain yogurts

Consume with moderation because they contain carbohydrates.

Nuts and oilseeds

They have low levels of carbohydrates, but are rich in saturated fatty acids, that's why they should moderate their consumption. Choose almonds, hazelnuts, Brazil nuts or pecans.

Coconut (in oil, cream or milk)

It contains saturated fatty acids, that's why we limit its consumption. Cream and coconut oil contain a lot of medium chain triglycerides (MCTs), which increase the level of ketones, essential to stay in ketosis.

Berries and red fruits

They contain carbohydrates, in reasonable quantities, but you should not abuse them to avoid ketosis (blueberries, blackberries, raspberries...).

9

Foods Allowed in Keto Diet

KETO-FRIENDLY
foods list.

FOODS

- Canned cod liver oil
- Canned tuna & salmon
- Canned sardines
- Free range organic eggs
- Fermented pickles
- Kimchi & sauerkraut
- Water buffalo yogurt
- Grassfed or raw cheeses
- Assorted nut butters
- Bone Broth - Chicken, beef or bison
- Low carb granola
- Musli
- Konjac noodles, spaghetti & rice
- Kelp noodles
- Shirataki noodles
- Local grassfed & grass finished meat
- Coconut wraps

SNACKS

- Meat sticks
- Local smoked oysters
- Crackers
- Pork crisps
- Macadamia nuts
- Seaweed snacks
- Coconut chips
- Sprouted pumpkin seeds
- Sprouted almonds
- Hemp hearts & seeds
- Low carb gummy bears
- Kale chips
- Ketone bars
- Collagen bars
- Low-carb protein bars
- Sugar free chocolate bars
- Low carb chocolate bars

DRINKS

- Kevita Lemon Cayenne
- Cold brew coffee
- Instant ketogenic coffee, tea, hot chocolate
- Coffee creamer

SAUCES

- Assorted avocado oil mayos
- Assorted avocado oil dressings
- Tomato sauce
- Sugar-free BBQ sauce
- No added sugar ketchup
- Zero carb mustard
- Guacamole
- Sour cream
- Pesto
- Siracha sauce
- Miso paste

FATS

- Beef tallow
- Pork lard
- Rendered duck fat
- Grassfed butter
- Ghee
- Coconut oil
- Raw coconut butter
- Coconut milk
- Coconut cream
- MCT oil
- Emulsified MCT oil
- Biodynamic olive oil
- Red palm oil
- Pure caprylic acid

BAKING

- Almond flour
- Coconut flour
- Monk fruit sweetener
- Organic stevia
- Baking chocolate
- Gelatin
- MCT powder
- Coconut milk powder
- Sugar-free chocolate chips

SUPPLEMENTS

- Instant ketones
- Brain Octane
- Collagen & gelatin
- L-Carnitine
- Magnesium
- Berberine
- Electrolyte liquid & powder
- Bone broth protein powder

I've had people complain about the difficulty of switching their grocery list to one that's Keto-genic-friendly. The fact is that food is expensive – and most of the food you have in your fridge are probably packed full with carbohydrates. This is why if you're committing to a Ketogenic Diet, you need to do a clean sweep. That's right – everything that's packed with carbohydrates should be identified and set aside to make sure you're not eating more than you should. You can donate them to a charity before going out and buying your new Keto-friendly shopping list.

Seafood

Seafood means fish like sardines, mackerel, and wild salmon. It's also a good idea to add some shrimp, tuna, mussels, and crab into your diet. This is going to be a tad expensive but definitely worth it in the long run. What's the common denominator in all these food items? The secret is omega-3 fatty acids which is credited for lots of health benefits. You want to add food rich in omega-3 fatty acids in your diet.

Low-carb Vegetables

Not all vegetables are good for you when it comes to the Ketogenic Diet. The vegetable choices should be limited to those with low carbohydrate counts. Pack up your cart with items like spinach, eggplant, arugula, broccoli, and cauliflower. You can also put in bell peppers, cabbage, celery, kale, Brussels sprouts, mushrooms, zucchini, and fennel.

So what's in them? Well, aside from the fact that they're low-carb, these vegetable also contain loads of fiber which makes digestion easier. Of course, there's also the presence of vitamins, minerals, antioxidants, and various other nutrients that you need for day to day life. Which ones should you avoid? Steer clear of the starch-packed vegetables like carrots, turnips, and beets. As a rule, you go for the vegetables that are green and leafy.

Fruits Low in Sugar

During an episode of sugar-craving, it's usually a good idea to pick low-sugar fruit items. Believe it or not, there are lots of those in the market! Just make sure to stock up on any of these: avocado, blackberries, raspberries, strawberries, blueberries, lime, lemon, and coconut. Also note that tomatoes are fruits too so feel free to make side dishes or dips with loads of tomatoes! Keep in mind that these fruits should be eaten fresh and not out of a can. If you do eat them fresh off the can however, take a good look at the nutritional information at the back of the packaging. Avocadoes are particularly popular for those practicing the Ketogenic Diet because they contains LOTS of the good kind of fat.

Meat and Eggs

While some diets will tell you to skip the meat, the Ketogenic Diet actually encourages its consumption. Meat is packed with protein that will feed your muscles and give you a consistent source of energy through the day. It's a slow but sure burn when you eat protein as opposed to carbohydrates which are burned faster and therefore stored faster if you don't use them immediately.

But what kind of meat should you be eating? There's chicken, beef, pork, venison, turkey, and lamb. Keep in mind that quality plays a huge role here – you should be eating grass-fed organic beef or organic poultry if you want to make the most out of this food variety. The organic option lets you limit the possibility of ingesting toxins in your body due to the production process of these products. Plus, the preservation process also means there are added salt or sugar in the meat, which can throw off the whole diet.

Nuts and Seeds

Nuts and seeds you should definitely add in your cart include: chia seeds, Brazil nuts, macadamia nuts, flaxseed, walnuts, hemp seeds, pecans, sesame seeds, almonds, hazelnut, and pumpkin seeds. They also contain lots of protein and very little sugar so they're great if you have the munchies. They're the ideal snack because they're quick, easy, and will keep you full. They're high in calories though, which is why lots of people steer clear of them. As I mentioned earlier though – the Ketogenic Diet has nothing to do with calories and everything to do with the nutrient you're eating. So don't pay too much attention on the calorie count and just remember that they're a good source of fats and protein.

Dairy Products

OK – some people in their 50s already have a hard time processing dairy products, but for those who don't – you can happily add many of these to your diet. Make sure to consume sufficient amounts of cheese, plain Greek yogurt, cream butter, and cottage cheese. These dairy products are packed with calcium, protein, and the healthy kind of fat.

Oils

Nope, we're not talking about essentials oils but rather, MCT oil, coconut oil, avocado oil, nut oils, and even extra-virgin olive oil. You can start using those for your frying needs to create healthier food options. The beauty of these oils is that they add flavor to the food, making sure you don't get bored quickly with the recipes. Try picking up different types of Keto-friendly oils to add some variety to your cooking.

Coffee and Tea

The good news is that you don't have to skip coffee if you're going on a Ketogenic Diet. The bad news is that you can't go to Starbucks anymore and order their blended coffee choices. Instead, beverages would be limited to unsweetened tea or unsweetened coffee in order to keep the sugar consumption low. Opt for organic coffee and tea products to make the most out of these powerful antioxidants.

Dark Chocolate

Yes – chocolate is still on the menu, but it is limited to just dark chocolate. Technically, this means eating chocolate that is 70 percent cacao, which would make the taste a bit bitter.

Sugar Substitutes

Later in the recipes part of this book, you might be surprised at some of the ingredients required in the list. This is because while sweeteners are an important part of food preparation, you can't just use any kind of sugar in your recipe. Remember: the typical sugar is pure carbohydrate. Even if you're not eating carbohydrates, if you're dumping lots of sugar in your food – you're not really following the Ketogenic Diet principles.

So what do you do? You find sugar substitutes. The good news is that there are LOTS of those in the market. You can get rid of the old sugar and use any of these as a good substitute.

Stevia. This is perhaps the most familiar one in this list. It's a natural sweetener derived from plants and contains very few calories. Unlike your typical sugar, stevia may actually help lower the sugar levels instead of causing it to spike. Note though that it's sweeter than actual sugar so when cooking with stevia, you'll need to lower the amount used. Typically, the ratio is 200 grams of sugar per 1 teaspoon of powdered stevia.

Sucralose. It contains zero calories and zero carbohydrates. It's actually an artificial sweetener and does not metabolize – hence the complete lack of carbohydrates. Splenda is actually a sweetener derived from sucralose. Note though that you don't want to use this as a baking substitute for sugar. Its best use is for coffee, yogurt, and oatmeal sweetening. Note though that like stevia, it's also very sweet – in fact, it's actually 600 times sweeter than the typical sugar. Use sparingly.

Erythritol. It's a naturally occurring compound that interacts with the tongue's sweet taste receptors. Hence, it mimics the taste of sugar without actually being sugar. It does contain calories, but only about 5% of the calories you'll find in the typical sugar. Note though that it doesn't dissolve very well so anything prepared with this sweetener will have a gritty feeling. This can be problematic if you're using the product for baking. As for sweetness, the typical ratio is 1 1/3 cup for 1 cup of sugar.

Xylitol. Like erythritol, xylitol is a type of sugar alcohol that's commonly used in sugar-free gum. While it still contains calories, the calories are just 3 per gram. It's a sweetener that's good for diabetic patients because it doesn't raise the sugar levels or insulin in the body. The great thing about this is that you don't have to do any computations when using it for baking, cooking, or fixing a drink. The ratio of it with sugar is 1 to 1 so you can quickly make the substitution in the recipe.

What about Condiments?

Condiments are still on the table, but they won't be as tasty as you're used to. Your options include mustard, olive oil mayonnaise, oil-based salad dressings, and unsweetened ketchup. Of all these condiments, ketchup is the one with the most sugar, so make a point of looking for one with reduced sugar content. Or maybe avoid ketchup altogether and stick to mustard?

What about Snacks?

The good news is that there are packed snacks for those who don't have the time to make it themselves. Sugarless nut butters, dried seaweeds, nuts, and sugar-free jerky are all available in stores. The nuts and seeds discussed in a previous paragraph all make for excellent snack options.

What about Labels?

Let's not fool ourselves into thinking that we can cook food every single day. The fact is that there will be days when there will be purchases for the sake of convenience. There are also instances when you'll have problems finding the right ingredients for a given recipe. Hence, you'll need to find substitutes for certain ingredients without losing the "Keto friendly" vibe of the product.

So what should be done? Well, you need to learn how to read labels. Food doesn't have to be specially made to be keto-friendly, you just have to make sure that it doesn't contain any of the unfriendly nutrients or that the carbohydrate content is low enough.

Salmon with Red Curry Sauce

Preparation Time: 10 minutes
Cooking Time: 22 minutes
Servings: 4
Ingredients:

- 4 salmon fillets
- 2 tablespoons olive oil
- Salt and pepper to taste
- 1 ½ tablespoons red curry paste
- 1 tablespoon fresh ginger, chopped
- 14 oz. coconut cream
- 1 ½ tablespoons fish sauce

Directions:

1. Preheat your oven to 350 degrees F.
2. Cover baking sheet with foil.
3. Brush both sides of salmon fillets with olive oil and season with salt and pepper.
4. Place the salmon fillets on the baking sheet.
5. Bake salmon in the oven for 20 minutes.
6. In a pan over medium heat, mix the curry paste, ginger, coconut cream and fish sauce.
7. Sprinkle with salt and pepper.
8. Simmer for 2 minutes.
9. Pour the sauce over the salmon before serving.

Nutrition:
Calories 553
Total Fat 43.4g
Saturated Fat 24.1g
Cholesterol 78mg
Sodium 908mg

Total Carbohydrate 7.9g
Dietary Fiber 2.4g
Total Sugars 3.6g
Protein 37.3g
Potassium 982mg

Salmon Teriyaki

Preparation Time: 15 minutes
Cooking Time: 25 minutes
Servings: 6
Ingredients:

- 3 tablespoons sesame oil
- 2 teaspoons fish sauce
- 3 tablespoons coconut amino
- 2 teaspoons ginger, grated
- 4 cloves garlic, crushed
- 2 tablespoons xylitol
- 1 tablespoon green lime juice
- 2 teaspoons green lime zest
- Cayenne pepper to taste
- 6 salmon fillets
- 1 teaspoon arrowroot starch
- ¼ cup water
- Sesame seeds

Directions:

1. Preheat your oven to 400 degrees F.
2. Combine the sesame oil, fish sauce, coconut amino, ginger, garlic, xylitol, green lime juice, zest and cayenne pepper in a mixing bowl.
3. Create 6 packets using foil.
4. Add half of the marinade in the packets.
5. Add the salmon inside.
6. Place in the baking sheet and cook for about 20 to 25 minutes.
7. Add the remaining sauce in a pan over medium heat.
8. Dissolve arrowroot in water, and add to the sauce.
9. Simmer until the sauce has thickened.

10. Place the salmon on a serving platter and pour the sauce on top.

11. Sprinkle sesame seeds on top before serving.

Nutrition:
Calories 312
Total Fat 17.9g
Saturated Fat 2.6g
Cholesterol 78mg
Sodium 242mg
Total Carbohydrate 3.5g
Dietary Fiber 0.1g
Total Sugars 0.1g
Protein 34.8g
Potassium 706mg

Pesto Shrimp with Zucchini Noodles

Preparation Time: 10 minutes
Cooking Time: 15 minutes
Servings: 3
Ingredients:

- Pesto sauce
- 3 cups basil leaves
- ¾ cup pine nuts
- 2 cloves garlic
- ½ lemon, juiced
- 1 teaspoon lemon zest
- Salt to taste
- ¼ cup olive oil
- Shrimp and Zoodles
- 3 zucchinis
- Salt to taste
- 1 lb. shrimp
- 2 tablespoons avocado oil

Directions:

1. Put all the pesto ingredients in a blender.
2. Blend until smooth.
3. Spiralize the zucchini into noodle form.
4. Season with salt.
5. Drain water from the zucchini noodles.
6. Season the shrimp with salt and pepper.
7. Add half of the oil in a pan over medium heat.
8. Once the oil is hot, add the shrimp and cook for 1 to 2 minutes.
9. Add the remaining oil to the pan.
10. Add the zucchini noodles and cook for 3 minutes.

11. Add the pesto and toss to coat the noodles evenly with the sauce.
12. Season with salt.

Nutrition:
Calories 304
Total Fat 22.2g
Saturated Fat 2.6g
Cholesterol 159mg
Sodium 223mg
Total Carbohydrate 8g
Dietary Fiber 2.3g
Total Sugars 2.5g
Protein 21.3g
Potassium 547mg

Crab Cakes

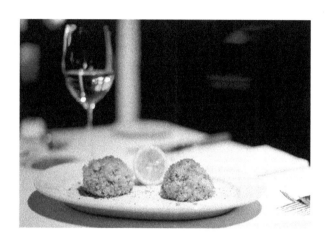

Preparation Time: 1 hour and 20 minutes
Cooking Time: 20 minutes
Servings: 8
Ingredients:

- 2 tablespoons butter
- 2 cloves garlic, minced
- ½ cup bell pepper, chopped
- 1 rib celery, chopped
- 1 shallot, chopped
- Salt and pepper to taste
- 2 tablespoons mayonnaise
- 1 egg, beaten
- 1 teaspoon mustard
- 1 tablespoon Worcestershire sauce
- 1 teaspoon hot sauce
- ½ cup Parmesan cheese, grated
- ½ cup pork rinds, crushed
- 1 lb. crabmeat
- 2 tablespoons olive oil

Directions:

- Add the butter to the pan over medium heat.
- Add the garlic, bell pepper, celery, shallot, salt and pepper.
- Cook for 10 minutes.
- In a bowl, mix the mayo, egg, Worcestershire, mustard and hot sauce.
- Add the sautéed vegetables to this mixture.
- Mix well.
- Add the cheese and pork rind.
- Fold in the crabmeat.
- Line the baking sheet with foil.
- Create patties from the mixture.
- Place the patties on the baking sheet.
- Cover the baking sheet with foil.
- Refrigerate for 1 hour.
- Fry in olive oil in a pan over medium heat.
- Cook until crispy and golden brown.

Nutrition:
Calories 150
Total Fat 9.2g
Saturated Fat 3.2g
Cholesterol 43mg
Sodium 601mg
Total Carbohydrate 10.8g
Dietary Fiber 0.5g
Total Sugars 4.6g
Protein 6.4g
Potassium 80mg

Tuna Salad

Preparation Time: 5 minutes
Cooking Time: 0 minute
Servings: 2
Ingredients:

- 1 cup tuna flakes
- 3 tablespoons mayonnaise
- 1 teaspoon onion flakes
- Salt and pepper to taste
- 3 cups Romaine lettuce

Directions:

1. Mix the tuna flakes, mayonnaise, onion flakes, salt and pepper in a bowl.
2. Serve with lettuce.

Nutrition:
Calories 130
Total Fat 7.8g
Saturated Fat 1.1g
Cholesterol 13mg
Sodium 206mg
Total Carbohydrate 8.5g
Dietary Fiber 0.6g
Total Sugars 2.6g
Protein 8.2g
Potassium 132mg

Keto Frosty

Preparation Time: 45 minutes
Cooking Time: 0 minute
Servings: 4
Ingredients:

- 1 ½ cups heavy whipping cream
- 2 tablespoons cocoa powder (unsweetened)
- 3 tablespoons Swerve
- 1 teaspoon pure vanilla extract
- Salt to taste

Directions:

1. In a bowl, combine all the ingredients.
2. Use a hand mixer and beat until you see stiff peaks forming.
3. Place the mixture in a Ziploc bag.
4. Freeze for 35 minutes.
5. Serve in bowls or dishes.

Nutrition:
Calories 164
Total Fat 17g
Saturated Fat 10.6g
Cholesterol 62mg
Sodium 56mg
Total Carbohydrate 2.9g
Dietary Fiber 0.8g
Total Sugars 0.2g
Protein 1.4g
Potassium 103mg

Keto Shake

Preparation Time: 15 minutes
Cooking Time: 0 minute
Serving: 1
Ingredients:

- ¾ cup almond milk
- ½ cup ice
- 2 tablespoons almond butter
- 2 tablespoons cocoa powder (unsweetened)
- 2 tablespoons Swerve
- 1 tablespoon chia seeds
- 2 tablespoons hemp seeds
- ½ tablespoon vanilla extract
- Salt to taste

Directions:

1. Blend all the ingredients in a food processor.
2. Chill in the refrigerator before serving.

Nutrition:
Calories 104
Total Fat 9.5g
Saturated Fat 5.1g
Cholesterol 0mg
Sodium 24mg
Total Carbohydrate 3.6g
Dietary Fiber 1.4g
Total Sugars 1.1g
Protein 2.9g
Potassium 159mg

Keto Fat Bombs

Preparation Time: 30 minutes
Cooking Time: 0 minute
Servings: 10
Ingredients:

- 8 tablespoons butter
- ¼ cup Swerve
- ½ teaspoon vanilla extract
- Salt to taste
- 2 cups almond flour
- 2/3 cup chocolate chips

Directions:

1. In a bowl, beat the butter until fluffy.
2. Stir in the sugar, salt and vanilla.
3. Mix well.
4. Add the almond flour.
5. Fold in the chocolate chips.
6. Cover the bowl with cling wrap and refrigerate for 20 minutes.
7. Create balls from the dough.

Nutrition:
Calories 176
Total Fat 15.2g
Saturated Fat 8.4g
Cholesterol 27mg
Sodium 92mg
Total Carbohydrate 12.9g
Dietary Fiber 1g
Total Sugars 10.8g

Protein 2.2g
Potassium 45mg

Avocado Ice Pops

Preparation Time: 20 minutes
Cooking Time: 0 minute
Servings: 10
Ingredients:

- 3 avocados
- ¼ cup lime juice
- 3 tablespoons Swerve
- ¾ cup coconut milk
- 1 tablespoon coconut oil
- 1 cup keto friendly chocolate

Directions:

1. Add all the ingredients except the oil and chocolate in a blender.
2. Blend until smooth.
3. Pour the mixture into the popsicle mold.
4. Freeze overnight.
5. In a bowl, mix oil and chocolate chips.
6. Melt in the microwave. And then let cool.
7. Dunk the avocado popsicles into the chocolate before serving.

Nutrition:
Calories 176
Total Fat 17.4g
Saturated Fat 7.5g
Cholesterol 0mg
Sodium 6mg
Total Carbohydrate 10.8g
Dietary Fiber 4.5g
Total Sugars 5.4g

Protein 1.6g
Potassium 341mg

Carrot Balls

Preparation Time: 1 hour and 10 minutes
Cooking Time: 0 minute
Servings: 8
Ingredients:

- 8 oz. block cream cheese
- ¾ cup coconut flour
- ½ teaspoon pure vanilla extract
- 1 teaspoon stevia
- ¼ teaspoon ground nutmeg
- 1 teaspoon cinnamon
- 1 cup carrots, grated
- 1/2 cup pecans, chopped
- 1 cup coconut, shredded

Directions:

Use a hand mixer to beat the cream cheese, coconut flour, vanilla, stevia, nutmeg and cinnamon.

Fold in the carrots and pecans.

Form into balls.

Refrigerate for 1 hour.

Roll into shredded coconut before serving.

Nutrition:
Calories 390
Total Fat 35g
Saturated Fat 17g
Cholesterol 60mg
Sodium 202mg
Total Carbohydrate 17.2g
Dietary Fiber 7.8g
Total Sugars 6g

Protein 7.8g
Potassium 154mg

Coconut Crack Bars

Preparation Time: 2 minutes
Cooking Time: 3 minutes
Servings: 20
Ingredients:

- 3 cups coconut flakes (unsweetened)
- 1 cup coconut oil
- ¼ cup maple syrup

Directions:

1. Line a baking sheet with parchment paper.
2. Put coconut in a bowl.
3. Add the oil and syrup.
4. Mix well.
5. Pour the mixture into the pan.
6. Refrigerate until firm.
7. Slice into bars before serving.

Nutrition:
Calories 147
Total Fat 14.9g
Saturated Fat 13g
Cholesterol 0mg
Sodium 3mg
Total Carbohydrate 4.5g
Dietary Fiber 1.1g
Total Sugars 3.1g
Protein 0.4g
Potassium 51mg

Strawberry Ice Cream

Preparation Time: 1 hour and 20 minutes
Cooking Time: 0 minute
Servings: 4
Ingredients:

- 17 oz. coconut milk
- 16 oz. frozen strawberries
- ¾ cup Swerve
- ½ cup fresh strawberries

Directions:

1. Put all the ingredients except fresh strawberries in a blender.
2. Pulse until smooth.
3. Put the mixture in an ice cream maker.
4. Use ice cream maker according to directions.
5. Add the fresh strawberries a few minutes before the ice cream is done.
6. Freeze for 1 hour before serving.

Nutrition:
Calories 320
Total Fat 28.8g
Saturated Fat 25.5g
Cholesterol 0mg
Sodium 18mg
Total Carbohydrate 25.3g
Dietary Fiber 5.3g
Total Sugars 19.1g
Protein 2.9g
Potassium 344mg

Key Lime Pudding

Preparation Time: 20 minutes
Cooking Time: 1 hour and 15 minutes
Servings: 2
Ingredients:

- 1 cup hot water
- 2/4 cup erythrytol syrup
- 6 drops stevia
- 1 teaspoon almond extract
- 1 teaspoon vanilla extract
- ¼ teaspoon Xanthan gum powder
- 2 ripe avocados, sliced
- 1 ½ oz. lime juice
- 3 tablespoons coconut oil
- Salt to taste

Directions:

1. Add water, erythritol, stevia, almond extract and vanilla extract to a pot.
2. Bring to a boil.
3. Simmer until the syrup has been reduced and has thickened.
4. Turn the heat off.
5. Add the gum powder.
6. Mix until thickened.
7. Add the avocado into a food processor.
8. Add the rest of the ingredients.
9. Pulse until smooth.
10. Place the mixture in ramekins.
11. Refrigerate for 1 hour.
12. Pour the syrup over the pudding before serving.

Nutrition:
Calories 299
Total Fat 29.8g
Saturated Fat 12.9g
Cholesterol 0mg
Sodium 47mg
Total Carbohydrate 9.7g
Dietary Fiber 6.8g
Total Sugars 0.8g
Protein 2g
Potassium 502mg

Chicken, Bacon and Avocado Cloud Sandwiches

Preparation Time: 10 minutes
Cooking Time: 25 minutes
Servings: 6
Ingredients:

- For cloud bread
- 3 large eggs
- 4 oz. cream cheese
- ½ tablespoon. ground psyllium husk powder
- ½ teaspoon baking powder
- A pinch of salt
- To assemble sandwich
- 6 slices of bacon, cooked and chopped
- 6 slices pepper Jack cheese
- ½ avocado, sliced
- 1 cup cooked chicken breasts, shredded
- 3 tablespoons. mayonnaise

Directions:

1. Preheat your oven to 300 degrees.
2. Prepare a baking sheet by lining it with parchment paper.
3. Separate the egg whites and egg yolks, and place into separate bowls.
4. Whisk the egg whites until very stiff. Set aside.
5. Combined egg yolks and cream cheese.
6. Add the psyllium husk powder and baking powder to the egg yolk mixture. Gently fold in.
7. Add the egg whites into the egg mixture and gently fold in.
8. Dollop the mixture onto the prepared baking sheet to create 12 cloud bread. Use a spatula to gently spread the circles around to form ½-inch thick pieces.
9. Bake for 25 minutes or until the tops are golden brown.

10. Allow the cloud bread to cool completely before serving. Can be refrigerated for up to 3 days of frozen for up to 3 months. If food prepping, place a layer of parchment paper between each bread slice to avoid having them getting stuck together. Simply toast in the oven for 5 minutes when it is time to serve.

11. To assemble sandwiches, place mayonnaise on one side of one cloud bread. Layer with the remaining sandwich ingredients and top with another slice of cloud bread.

Nutrition:
Calories: 333 kcal
Carbs: 5g
Fat: 26g
Protein: 19.9g

Roasted Lemon Chicken Sandwich

Preparation Time: 15 minutes
Cooking Time: 1 hour 30 minutes
Servings: 12
Ingredients:

- 1 kg whole chicken
- 5 tablespoons. butter
- 1 lemon, cut into wedges
- 1 tablespoon. garlic powder

- Salt and pepper to taste
- 2 tablespoons. mayonnaise
- Keto-friendly bread

Directions:

1. Preheat the oven to 350 degrees F.
2. Grease a deep baking dish with butter.
3. Ensure that the chicken is patted dry and that the gizzards have been removed.
4. Combine the butter, garlic powder, salt and pepper.
5. Rub the entire chicken with it, including in the cavity.
6. Place the lemon and onion inside the chicken and place the chicken in the prepared baking dish.
7. Bake for about 1½ hours, depending on the size of the chicken.
8. Baste the chicken often with the drippings. If the drippings begin to dry, add water. The chicken is done when a thermometer, insert it into the thickest part of the thigh reads 165 degrees F or when the clear juices run when the thickest part of the thigh is pierced.
9. Allow the chicken to cool before slicing.
10. To assemble sandwich, shred some of the breast meat and mix with the mayonnaise. Place the mixture between the two bread slices.
11. To save the chicken, refrigerated for up to 5 days or freeze for up to 1 month.

Nutrition:
Calories: 214 kcal
Carbs: 1.6 g
Fat: 11.8 g
Protein: 24.4 g.

Keto-Friendly Skillet Pepperoni Pizza

Preparation Time: 10 minutes
Cooking Time: 6 minutes
Servings: 4
Ingredients:
For Crust
½ cup almond flour
½ teaspoon baking powder
8 large egg whites, whisked into stiff peaks
Salt and pepper to taste
Toppings
3 tablespoons. Unsweetened tomato sauce
½ cup shredded cheddar cheese
½ cup pepperoni
Directions
Gently incorporate the almond flour into the egg whites. Ensure that no lumps remain.
Stir in the remaining crust ingredients.
Heat a nonstick skillet over medium heat. Spray with nonstick spray.
Pour the batter into the heated skillet to cover the bottom of the skillet.
Cover the skillet with a lid and cook the pizza crust to cook for about 4 minutes or until bubbles that appear on the top.
Flip the dough and add the toppings, starting with the tomato sauce and ending with the pepperoni
Cook the pizza for 2 more minutes.
Allow the pizza to cool slightly before serving.
Can be stored in the refrigerator for up to 5 days and frozen for up to 1 month.
Nutrition:
Calories: 175 kcal
Carbs: 1.9 g
Fat: 12 g
Protein: 14.3 g.

Cheesy Chicken Cauliflower

Preparation Time: 5 minutes
Cooking Time: 10 minutes
Servings: 4
Ingredients:

- 2 cups cauliflower florets, chopped
- ½ cup red bell pepper, chopped
- 1 cup roasted chicken, shredded (Lunch Recipes: Roasted Lemon Chicken Sandwich)
- ¼ cup shredded cheddar cheese
- 1 tablespoon. butter
- 1 tablespoon. sour cream
- Salt and pepper to taste

Directions:

1. Stir fry the cauliflower and peppers in the butter over medium heat until the veggies are tender.
2. Add the chicken and cook until the chicken is warmed through.
3. Add the remaining ingredients and stir until the cheese is melted.
4. Serve warm.

Nutrition:
Calories: 144 kcal
Carbs: 4 g
Fat: 8.5 g
Protein: 13.2 g.

Chicken Soup

Preparation Time: 10 minutes
Cooking Time: 25 minutes
Servings: 6
Ingredients:

- 4 cups roasted chicken, shredded (Lunch Recipes: Roasted Lemon Chicken Sandwich)
- 2 tablespoons. butter
- 2 celery stalks, chopped
- 1 cup mushrooms, sliced
- 4 cups green cabbage, sliced into strips
- 2 garlic cloves, minced
- 6 cups chicken broth
- 1 carrot, sliced
- Salt and pepper to taste
- 1 tablespoon. garlic powder
- 1 tablespoon. onion powder

Directions:

1. Sauté the celery, mushrooms and garlic in the butter in a pot over medium heat for 4 minutes.
2. Add broth, carrots, garlic powder, onion powder, salt, and pepper.
3. Simmer for 10 minutes or until the vegetables are tender.
4. Add the chicken and cabbage and simmer for another 10 minutes or until the cabbage is tender.
5. Serve warm.
6. Can be refrigerated for up to 3 days or frozen for up to 1 month.

Nutrition:
Calories: 279 kcal
Carbs: 7.5 g
Fat: 12.3 g

Protein: 33.4 g.

Chicken Avocado Salad

Preparation Time: 7 minutes
Cooking Time: 10 minutes
Servings: 4
Ingredients:

- 1 cup roasted chicken, shredded (Lunch Recipes: Roasted Lemon Chicken Sandwich)
- 1 bacon strip, cooked and chopped
- 1/2 medium avocado, chopped
- ¼ cup cheddar cheese, grated
- 1 hard-boiled egg, chopped
- 1 cup romaine lettuce, chopped
- 1 tablespoon. olive oil
- 1 tablespoon. apple cider vinegar
- Salt and pepper to taste

Directions:

1. Create the dressing by mixing apple cider vinegar, oil, salt and pepper.
2. Combine all the other ingredients in a mixing bowl.
3. Drizzle with the dressing and toss.

4. Can be refrigerated for up to 3 days.

Nutrition:
Calories: 220 kcal
Carbs: 2.8 g
Fat: 16.7 g
Protein: 14.8 g.

Chicken Broccoli Dinner

Preparation Time: 10 minutes
Cooking Time: 5 minutes
Servings: 1
Ingredients:

- 1 roasted chicken leg (Lunch Recipes: Roasted Lemon Chicken Sandwich)
- ½ cup broccoli florets
- ½ tablespoon. unsalted butter, softened
- 2 garlic cloves, minced

- Salt and pepper to taste

Directions:

1. Boil the broccoli in lightly salted water for 5 minutes. Drain the water from the pot and keep the broccoli in the pot. Keep the lid on to keep the broccoli warm.
2. Mix all the butter, garlic, salt and pepper in a small bowl to create garlic butter.
3. Place the chicken, broccoli and garlic butter.

Nutrition:
Calories: 257 kcal
Carbs: 5.1 g
Fat: 14 g
Protein: 27.4 g.

Easy Meatballs

Preparation Time: 10 minutes
Cooking Time: 20 minutes
Servings: 4
Ingredients:

- 1 lb. ground beef
- 1 egg, beaten
- Salt and pepper to taste
- 1 teaspoon garlic powder
- 1 teaspoon onion powder
- 2 tablespoons. butter
- ¼ cup mayonnaise
- ¼ cup pickled jalapeños
- 1 cup cheddar cheese, grated

Directions

1. Combine the cheese, mayonnaise, pickled jalapenos, salt, pepper, garlic powder and onion powder in a large mixing bowl.
2. Add the beef and egg and combine using clean hands.
3. Form large meatballs. Makes about 12.
4. Fry the meatballs in the butter over medium heat for about 4 minutes on each side or until golden brown.
5. Serve warm with a keto-friendly side.
6. The meatball mixture can also be used to make a meatloaf. Just preheat your oven to 400 degrees F, press the mixture into a loaf pan and bake for about 30 minutes or until the top is golden brown.
7. Can be refrigerated for up to 5 days or frozen for up to 3 months.

Nutrition:
Calories: 454 kcal

Carbs: 5 g
Fat: 28.2 g
Protein: 43.2 g.

Chicken Casserole

Preparation Time: 10 minutes
Cooking Time: 40 minutes
Servings: 8
Ingredients:

- 1 lb. boneless chicken breasts, cut into 1" cubes
- 2 tablespoons. butter
- 4 tablespoons. green pesto
- 1 cup heavy whipping cream
- ¼ cup green bell peppers, diced
- 1 cup feta cheese, diced
- 1 garlic clove, minced
- Salt and pepper to taste

Directions

1. Preheat your oven to 400 degrees F.
2. Season the chicken with salt and pepper then batch fry in the butter until golden brown.
3. Place the fried chicken pieces in a baking dish. Add the feta cheese, garlic and bell peppers.
4. Combine the pesto and heavy cream in a bowl. Pour on top of the chicken mixture and spread with a spatula.
5. Bake for 30 minutes or until the casserole is light brown around the edges.
6. Serve warm.
7. Can be refrigerated for up to 5 days and frozen for 2 weeks.

Nutrition:
Calories: 294 kcal
Carbs: 1.7 g
Fat: 22.7 g
Protein: 20.1 g.

Lemon Baked Salmon

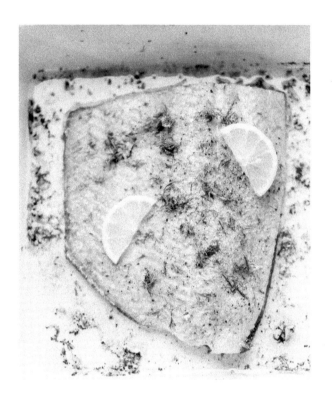

Preparation Time: 10 minutes
Cooking Time: 30 minutes
Servings: 4
Ingredients:

- 1 lb. salmon
- 1 tablespoon. olive oil
- Salt and pepper to taste
- 1 tablespoon. butter
- 1 lemon, thinly sliced
- 1 tablespoon. lemon juice

Directions:

1. Preheat your oven to 400 degrees F.
2. Grease a baking dish with the olive oil and place the salmon skin-side down.
3. Season the salmon with salt and pepper then top with the lemon slices.
4. Slice half the butter and place over the salmon.
5. Bake for 20minutes or until the salmon flakes easily.
6. Melt the remaining butter in a saucepan. When it starts to bubble, remove from heat and allow to cool before adding the lemon juice.
7. Drizzle the lemon butter over the salmon and Serve warm.

Nutrition:
Calories: 211 kcal
Carbs: 1.5 g
Fat: 13.5 g
Protein: 22.2 g.

Italian Sausage Stacks

Preparation Time: 10 minutes
Cooking Time: 25 minutes
Servings: 3
Ingredients:

- 6 Italian sausage patties
- 4 tablespoon olive oil
- 2 ripe avocados, pitted
- 2 teaspoon fresh lime juice
- Salt and black pepper to taste
- 6 fresh eggs
- Red pepper flakes to garnish

Directions:

1. In a skillet, warm the oil over medium heat and fry the sausage patties about 8 minutes until lightly browned and firm. Remove the patties to a plate.
2. Spoon the avocado into a bowl, mash with the lime juice, and season with salt and black pepper. Spread the mash on the sausages.
3. Boil 3 cups of water in a wide pan over high heat, and reduce to simmer (don't boil).
4. Crack each egg into a small bowl and gently put the egg into the simmering water; poach for 2 to 3 minutes. Use a perforated spoon to remove from the water on a paper towel to dry. Repeat with the other 5 eggs. Top each stack with a poached egg, sprinkle with chili flakes, salt, black pepper, and chives. Serve with turnip wedges.

Nutrition:
Kcal 378,
Fat 23g,
Net Carbs 5g,
Protein 16g

Baked Salmon

Preparation Time: 10 minutes
Cooking Time: 10 minutes
Servings: 4
Ingredients:

- Cooking spray
- 3 cloves garlic, minced
- ¼ cup butter
- 1 teaspoon lemon zest
- 2 tablespoons lemon juice
- 4 salmon fillets
- Salt and pepper to taste
- 2 tablespoons parsley, chopped

Directions:

1. Preheat your oven to 425 degrees F.
2. Grease the pan with cooking spray.
3. In a bowl, mix the garlic, butter, and lemon zest and lemon juice.
4. Sprinkle salt and pepper on salmon fillets.
5. Drizzle with the lemon butter sauce.
6. Bake in the oven for 12 minutes.
7. Garnish with parsley before serving.

Nutrition:
Calories 345
Total Fat 22.7g
Saturated Fat 8.9g
Cholesterol 109mg
Sodium 163mg
Total Carbohydrate 1.2g

Dietary Fiber 0.2g
Total Sugars 0.2g
Protein 34.9g
Potassium 718mg

Tuna Patties

Preparation Time: 10 minutes
Cooking Time: 10 minutes
Servings: 8
Ingredients:

- 20 oz. canned tuna flakes
- ¼ cup almond flour
- 1 egg, beaten
- 2 tablespoons fresh dill, chopped
- 2 stalks green onion, chopped
- Salt and pepper to taste
- 1 tablespoon lemon zest
- ¼ cup mayonnaise
- 1 tablespoon lemon juice
- 2 tablespoons avocado oil

Directions:

1. Combine all the ingredients except avocado oil, lemon juice and avocado oil in a large bowl.
2. Form 8 patties from the mixture.
3. In a pan over medium heat, add the oil.

4. Once the oil starts to sizzle, cook the tuna patties for 3 to 4 minutes per side.

5. Drain each patty on a paper towel.

6. Spread mayo on top and drizzle with lemon juice before serving.

Nutrition:

Calories 101

Total Fat 4.9g

Saturated Fat 1.2g

Cholesterol 47mg

Sodium 243mg

Total Carbohydrate 3.1g

Dietary Fiber 0.5g

Total Sugars 0.7g

Protein 12.3g

Potassium 60mg

Cauliflower Mash

Preparation Time: 10 minutes
Cooking Time: 5 minutes
Servings: 8
Ingredients:

- 4 cups cauliflower florets, chopped
- 1 cup grated parmesan cheese
- 6 tablespoons. butter
- ½ lemon, juice and zest
- Salt and pepper to taste

Directions:

1. Boil the cauliflower in lightly salted water over high heat for 5 minutes or until the florets are tender but still firm.
2. Strain the cauliflower in a colander and add the cauliflower to a food processor
3. Add the remaining ingredients and pulse the mixture to a smooth and creamy consistency
4. Serve with protein like salmon, chicken or meatballs.
5. Can be refrigerated for up to 3 days.

Nutrition:
Calories: 101 kcal
Carbs: 3.1 g
Fat: 9.5 g
Protein: 2.2 g.

Almond Waffles with Cinnamon Cream

Preparation Time: 10 minutes
Cooking Time: 25 minutes
Servings: 3
Ingredients:

- For the Spread
- 8 oz. cream cheese, at room temperature
- 1 teaspoon cinnamon powder
- 3 tablespoon swerve brown sugar
- Cinnamon powder for garnishing
- For the Waffles
- 5 tablespoon melted butter
- 1 ½ cups unsweetened almond milk
- 7 large eggs
- ¼ teaspoon liquid stevia
- ½ teaspoon baking powder
- 1 ½ cups almond flour

Directions:

1. Combine the cream cheese, cinnamon, and swerve with a hand mixer until smooth. Cover and chill until ready to use.
2. To make the waffles, whisk the butter, milk, and eggs in a medium bowl. Add the stevia and baking powder and mix. Stir in the almond flour and combine until no lumps exist. Let the batter sit for 5 minutes to thicken. Spritz a waffle iron with a non-stick cooking spray.
3. Ladle a ¼ cup of the batter into the waffle iron and cook according to the manufacturer's instructions until golden, about 10 minutes in total. Repeat with the remaining batter.
4. Slice the waffles into quarters; apply the cinnamon spread in between each of two waffles and snap. Sprinkle with cinnamon powder and serve.

Nutrition:

Kcal 307,
Fat 24g,
Net Carbs 8g,
Protein 12g

Grilled Mahi with Lemon Butter Sauce

Preparation Time: 20 minutes
Cooking Time: 10 minutes
Servings: 6
Ingredients:

- 6 mahi fillets
- Salt and pepper to taste
- 2 tablespoons olive oil
- 6 tablespoons butter
- ¼ onion, minced
- ½ teaspoon garlic, minced
- ¼ cup chicken stock
- 1 tablespoon lemon juice

Directions:

1. Preheat your grill to medium heat.
2. Season fish fillets with salt and pepper.
3. Coat both sides with olive oil.
4. Grill for 3 to 4 minutes per side.
5. Place fish on a serving platter.
6. In a pan over medium heat, add the butter and let it melt.
7. Add the onion and sauté for 2 minutes.
8. Add the garlic and cook for 30 seconds.
9. Pour in the chicken stock.
10. Simmer until the stock has been reduced to half.
11. Add the lemon juice.
12. Pour the sauce over the grilled fish fillets.

Nutrition:
Calories 234

Total Fat 17.2g
Saturated Fat 8.3g
Cholesterol 117mg
Sodium 242mg
Total Carbohydrate 0.6g
Dietary Fiber 0.1g
Total Sugars 0.3g
Protein 19.1g
Potassium 385mg

Shrimp Scampi

Preparation Time: 15 minutes
Cooking Time: 10 minutes
Servings: 6
Ingredients:

- 2 tablespoons olive oil
- 2 tablespoons butter
- 1 tablespoon garlic, minced
- ½ cup dry white wine
- ¼ teaspoon red pepper flakes
- Salt and pepper to taste
- 2 lb. large shrimp, peeled and deveined
- ¼ cup fresh parsley, chopped
- 1 teaspoon lemon zest
- 2 tablespoons lemon juice
- 3 cups spaghetti squash, cooked

Directions:

1. In a pan over medium heat, add the oil and butter.
2. Cook the garlic for 2 minutes.

3. Pour in the wine.
4. Add the red pepper flakes, salt and pepper.
5. Cook for 2 minutes.
6. Add the shrimp.
7. Cook for 2 to 3 minutes.
8. Remove from the stove.
9. Add the parsley, lemon zest and lemon juice.
10. Serve on top of spaghetti squash.

Nutrition:
Calories 232
Total Fat 8.9g
Saturated Fat 3.2g
Cholesterol 226mg
Sodium 229mg
Total Carbohydrate 7.6g
Dietary Fiber 0.2g
Total Sugars 0.3g
Protein 28.9g
Potassium 104mg

Dark Chocolate Smoothie

Preparation Time: 10 minutes
Cooking Time: 25 minutes
Servings: 3
Ingredients:

- 8 pecans
- ¾ cup coconut milk
- ¼ cup water
- 1 ½ cups watercress
- 2 teaspoon vegan protein powder
- 1 tablespoon chia seeds
- 1 tablespoon unsweetened cocoa powder
- 4 fresh dates, pitted

Directions

1. In a blender, add all ingredients and process until creamy and uniform. Place into two glasses and chill before serving.

Nutrition:
Kcal 335;
Fat: 31.7g
Net Carbs: 12.7g,
Protein: 7g

Five Greens Smoothie

Preparation Time: 10 minutes
Cooking Time: 25 minutes
Servings: 3
Ingredients:

- 6 kale leaves, chopped
- 3 stalks celery, chopped
- 1 ripe avocado, skinned, pitted, sliced
- 1 cup ice cubes
- 2 cups spinach, chopped
- 1 large cucumber, peeled and chopped
- Chia seeds to garnish

Directions:

1. In a blender, add the kale, celery, avocado, and ice cubes, and blend for 45 seconds. Add the spinach and cucumber, and process for another 45 seconds until smooth.
2. Pour the smoothie into glasses, garnish with chia seeds and serve the drink immediately.

Nutrition:
Kcal 124,
Fat 7.8g,
Net Carbs 2.9g,
Protein 3.2g

Smoked Salmon Rolls with Dill Cream Cheese

Preparation Time: 10 minutes
Cooking Time: 25 minutes
Servings: 3
Ingredients:

- 3 tablespoon cream cheese, softened
- 1 small lemon, zested and juiced
- 3 teaspoon chopped fresh dill
- Salt and black pepper to taste
- 3 (7-inch) low carb tortillas
- 6 slices smoked salmon

Directions

1. In a bowl, mix the cream cheese, lemon juice, zest, dill, salt, and black pepper.
2. Lay each tortilla on a plastic wrap (just wide enough to cover the tortilla), spread with cream cheese mixture, and top each (one) with two salmon slices. Roll up the tortillas and secure both ends by twisting.
3. Refrigerate for 2 hours, remove plastic, cut off both ends of each wrap, and cut wraps into wheels.

Nutrition:
Kcal 250,
Fat 16g,
Net Carbs 7g,
Protein 18g

Pan-Seared Halibut with Citrus Butter Sauce

Preparation Time: 10 minutes
Cooking Time: 15 minutes
Servings: 3
Ingredients:

- 4 (5-ounce) halibut fillets, each about 1 inch thick
- Sea salt
- Freshly ground black pepper
- ¼ cup butter
- 2 teaspoons minced garlic
- 1 shallot, minced
- 3 tablespoons dry white wine
- 1 tablespoon freshly squeezed lemon juice
- 1 tablespoon freshly squeezed orange juice
- 2 teaspoons chopped fresh parsley
- 2 tablespoons olive oil

Directions:

1. Pat the fish dry with paper towels and then lightly season the fillets with salt and pepper. Set aside on a paper towel–lined plate.
2. Place a small saucepan over medium heat and melt the butter.
3. Sauté the garlic and shallot until tender, about 3 minutes.
4. Whisk in the white wine, lemon juice, and orange juice and bring the sauce to a simmer, cooking until it thickens slightly, about 2 minutes.
5. Remove the sauce from the heat and stir in the parsley; set aside.
6. Place a large skillet over medium-high heat and add the olive oil.
7. Panfry the fish until lightly browned and just cooked through, turning them over once, about 10 minutes in total.
8. Serve the fish immediately with a spoonful of sauce for each.

Nutrition:
Calories: 319
Fat: 26g
Protein: 22g
Carbohydrates: 2g
Fiber: 0g

Lemon Butter Chicken

Preparation Time: 10 minutes
Cooking Time: 40 minutes
Servings: 4
Ingredients:

- 4 bone-in, skin-on chicken thighs
- Sea salt
- Freshly ground black pepper
- 2 tablespoons butter, divided
- 2 teaspoons minced garlic
- ½ cup Herbed Chicken Stock
- ½ cup heavy (whipping) cream
- Juice of ½ lemon

Directions:

1. Preheat the oven to 400°F.
2. Lightly season the chicken thighs with salt and pepper.
3. Place a large ovenproof skillet over medium-high heat and add 1 tablespoon of butter.
4. Brown the chicken thighs until golden on both sides, about 6 minutes in total. Remove the thighs to a plate and set aside.
5. Add the remaining 1 tablespoon of butter and sauté the garlic until translucent, about 2 minutes.
6. Whisk in the chicken stock, heavy cream, and lemon juice.
7. Bring the sauce to a boil and then return the chicken to the skillet.
8. Place the skillet in the oven, covered, and braise until the chicken is cooked through, about 30 minutes.

Nutrition:
Calories: 294
Fat: 26g

Protein: 12g
Carbohydrates: 4g
Fiber: 1g

Simple Fish Curry

Preparation Time: 10 minutes
Cooking Time: 25 minutes
Servings: 4
Ingredients:

- 2 tablespoons coconut oil
- 1½ tablespoons grated fresh ginger
- 2 teaspoons minced garlic
- 1 tablespoon curry powder
- ½ teaspoon ground cumin
- 2 cups coconut milk
- 16 ounces firm white fish, cut into 1-inch chunks
- 1 cup shredded kale
- 2 tablespoons chopped cilantro

Directions:

1. Place a large saucepan over medium heat and melt the coconut oil.
2. Sauté the ginger and garlic until lightly browned, about 2 minutes.
3. Stir in the curry powder and cumin and sauté until very fragrant, about 2 minutes.
4. Stir in the coconut milk and bring the liquid to a boil.
5. Reduce the heat to low and simmer for about 5 minutes to infuse the milk with the spices.
6. Add the fish and cook until the fish is cooked through, about 10 minutes.
7. Stir in the kale and cilantro and simmer until wilted, about 2 minutes.
8. Serve.

Nutrition:
Calories: 416
Fat: 31g
Protein: 26g
Carbohydrates: 5g

Fiber: 1g]

Roasted Salmon with Avocado Salsa

Preparation Time: 15 minutes
Cooking Time: 12 minutes
Servings: 4
Ingredients:

- For the Salsa
- 1 avocado, peeled, pitted, and diced
- 1 scallion, white and green parts, chopped
- ½ cup halved cherry tomatoes
- Juice of 1 lemon
- Zest of 1 lemon
- For the Fish
- 1 teaspoon ground cumin
- ½ teaspoon ground coriander
- ½ teaspoon onion powder
- ¼ teaspoon sea salt
- Pinch freshly ground black pepper
- Pinch cayenne pepper
- 4 (4-ounce) boneless, skinless salmon fillets
- 2 tablespoons olive oil

Directions:

1. To Make the Salsa
2. In a small bowl, stir together the avocado, scallion, tomatoes, lemon juice, and lemon zest until mixed.
3. Set aside.
4. To Make the Fish
5. Preheat the oven to 400°F. Line a baking sheet with aluminum foil and set aside.
6. In a small bowl, stir together the cumin, coriander, onion powder, salt, black pepper, and cayenne until well mixed.

7. Rub the salmon fillets with the spice mix and place them on the baking sheet.

8. Drizzle the fillets with the olive oil and roast the fish until it is just cooked through, about 15 minutes.

9. Serve the salmon topped with the avocado salsa.

Nutrition:
Calories: 320
Fat: 26g
Protein: 22g
Carbohydrates: 4g
Fiber: 3g

Sole Asiago

Preparation Time: 10 minutes
Cooking Time: 8 minutes
Servings: 4
Ingredients:

- 4 (4-ounce) sole fillets
- ¾ cup ground almonds
- ¼ cup Asiago cheese
- 2 eggs, beaten
- 2½ tablespoons melted coconut oil

Directions:

1. Preheat the oven to 350°F. Line a baking sheet with parchment paper and set aside.
2. Pat the fish dry with paper towels.
3. Stir together the ground almonds and cheese in a small bowl.
4. Place the bowl with the beaten eggs in it next to the almond mixture.
5. Dredge a sole fillet in the beaten egg and then press the fish into the almond mixture so it is completely coated. Place on the baking sheet and repeat until all the fillets are breaded.
6. Brush both sides of each piece of fish with the coconut oil.
7. Bake the sole until it is cooked through, about 8 minutes in total.
8. Serve immediately.

Nutrition:
Calories: 406
Fat: 31g
Protein: 29g
Carbohydrates: 6g
Fiber: 3g

Baked Coconut Haddock

Preparation Time: 10 minutes
Cooking Time: 12 minutes
Servings: 4
Ingredients:

- 4 (5-ounce) boneless haddock fillets
- Sea salt
- Freshly ground black pepper
- 1 cup shredded unsweetened coconut
- ¼ cup ground hazelnuts
- 2 tablespoons coconut oil, melted

Directions:

1. Preheat the oven to 400°F. Line a baking sheet with parchment paper and set aside.
2. Pat the fillets very dry with paper towels and lightly season them with salt and pepper.
3. Stir together the shredded coconut and hazelnuts in a small bowl.
4. Dredge the fish fillets in the coconut mixture so that both sides of each piece are thickly coated.
5. Place the fish on the baking sheet and lightly brush both sides of each piece with the coconut oil.
6. Bake the haddock until the topping is golden and the fish flakes easily with a fork, about 12 minutes total.
7. Serve.
8. PREP TIP the breading of the fish can be done ahead, up to 1 day, if you just want to pop the fish in the oven when you get home. Place the breaded fish on the baking sheet and cover it with plastic wrap in the refrigerator until you wish to bake it.

Nutrition:
Calories: 299
Fat: 24g

Protein: 20g
Carbohydrates: 4g
Fiber: 3g

Cheesy Garlic Salmon

Preparation Time: 15 minutes
Cooking Time: 12 minutes
Servings: 4
Ingredients:

- ½ cup Asiago cheese
- 2 tablespoons freshly squeezed lemon juice
- 2 tablespoons butter, at room temperature
- 2 teaspoons minced garlic
- 1 teaspoon chopped fresh basil
- 1 teaspoon chopped fresh oregano
- 4 (5-ounce) salmon fillets
- 1 tablespoon olive oil

Directions:

1. Preheat the oven to 350°F. Line a baking sheet with parchment paper and set aside.
2. In a small bowl, stir together the Asiago cheese, lemon juice, butter, garlic, basil, and oregano.
3. Pat the salmon dry with paper towels and place the fillets on the baking sheet skin-side down. Divide the topping evenly between the fillets and spread it across the fish using a knife or the back of a spoon.
4. Drizzle the fish with the olive oil and bake until the topping is golden and the fish is just cooked through, about 12 minutes.
5. Serve.

Nutrition:
Calories: 357
Fat: 28g
Protein: 24g
Carbohydrates: 2g
Fiber: 0g

Chicken Bacon Burgers

Preparation Time: 10 minutes
Cooking Time: 25 minutes
Servings: 4
Ingredients:

- 1-pound ground chicken
- 8 bacon slices, chopped
- ¼ cup ground almonds
- 1 teaspoon chopped fresh basil
- ¼ teaspoon sea salt
- Pinch freshly ground black pepper
- 2 tablespoons coconut oil
- 4 large lettuce leaves
- 1 avocado, peeled, pitted, and sliced

Directions:

1. Preheat the oven to 350°F. Line a baking sheet with parchment paper and set aside.
2. In a medium bowl, combine the chicken, bacon, ground almonds, basil, salt, and pepper until well mixed.
3. Form the mixture into 6 equal patties.
4. Place a large skillet over medium-high heat and add the coconut oil.
5. Pan sear the chicken patties until brown on both sides, about 6 minutes in total.
6. Place the browned patties on the baking sheet and bake until completely cooked through, about 15 minutes.
7. Serve on the lettuce leaves, topped with the avocado slices.

Nutrition:
Calories: 374
Fat: 33g
Protein: 18g

Carbohydrates: 3g
Fiber: 2g

Herb Butter Scallops

Preparation Time: 10 minutes
Cooking Time: 10 minutes
Servings: 3
Ingredients:

- 1 pound sea scallops, cleaned
- Freshly ground black pepper
- 8 tablespoons butter, divided
- 2 teaspoons minced garlic
- Juice of 1 lemon
- 2 teaspoons chopped fresh basil
- 1 teaspoon chopped fresh thyme

Directions:

1. Pat the scallops dry with paper towels and season them lightly with pepper.
2. Place a large skillet over medium heat and add 2 tablespoons of butter.
3. Arrange the scallops in the skillet, evenly spaced but not too close together, and sear each side until they are golden brown, about 2½ minutes per side.
4. Remove the scallops to a plate and set aside.
5. Add the remaining 6 tablespoons of butter to the skillet and sauté the garlic until translucent, about 3 minutes.
6. Stir in the lemon juice, basil, and thyme and return the scallops to the skillet, turning to coat them in the sauce.
7. Serve immediately.

Nutrition:
Calories: 306
Fat: 24g
Protein: 19g
Carbohydrates: 4g

Fiber: 0g

Paprika Chicken

Preparation Time: 10 minutes
Cooking Time: 25 minutes
Servings: 4
Ingredients:

- 4 (4-ounce) chicken breasts, skin-on
- Sea salt
- Freshly ground black pepper
- 1 tablespoon olive oil
- ½ cup chopped sweet onion
- ½ cup heavy (whipping) cream
- 2 teaspoons smoked paprika
- ½ cup sour cream
- 2 tablespoons chopped fresh parsley

Directions:

1. Lightly season the chicken with salt and pepper.
2. Place a large skillet over medium-high heat and add the olive oil.
3. Sear the chicken on both sides until almost cooked through, about 15 minutes in total. Remove the chicken to a plate.
4. Add the onion to the skillet and sauté until tender, about 4 minutes.
5. Stir in the cream and paprika and bring the liquid to a simmer.
6. Return the chicken and any accumulated juices to the skillet and simmer the chicken for 5 minutes until completely cooked.
7. Stir in the sour cream and remove the skillet from the heat.
8. Serve topped with the parsley.

Nutrition:
Calories: 389
Fat: 30g

Protein: 25g
Carbohydrates: 4g
Fiber: 0g

Trout and Chili Nuts

Preparation Time: 10 minutes
Cooking time: 0 minutes
Servings: 3
Ingredients:

- 1.5kg of rainbow trout
- 300gr shelled walnuts
- 1 bunch of parsley
- 9 cloves of garlic
- 7 tablespoons of olive oil
- 2 fresh hot peppers
- The juice of 2 lemons
- Halls

Directions:

1. Clean and dry the trout then place them in a baking tray.
2. Chop the walnuts, parsley and chili peppers then mash the garlic cloves.
3. Mix the ingredients by adding olive oil, lemon juice and a pinch of salt.
4. Stuff the trout with some of the sauce and use the rest to cover the fish.
5. Bake at 180° for 30/40 minutes.
6. Serve the trout hot or cold.

Nutrition:
Calories 226
Fat 5
Fiber 2
Carbs 7
Protein 8

Nut Granola & Smoothie Bowl

Preparation Time: 10 minutes
Cooking time: 40 minutes
Servings: 3
Ingredients:

- 6 cups Greek yogurt
- 4 tablespoon almond butter
- A handful toasted walnuts
- 3 tablespoon unsweetened cocoa powder
- 4 teaspoon swerve brown sugar
- 2 cups nut granola for topping

Directions:

1. Combine the Greek yogurt, almond butter, walnuts, cocoa powder, and swerve brown sugar in a smoothie maker; puree in high-speed until smooth and well mixed.
2. Share the smoothie into four breakfast bowls, top with a half cup of granola each, and serve.

Nutrition:
Kcal 361,
Fat 31.2g,
Net Carbs 2g,
Protein 13g

Bacon and Egg Quesadillas

Preparation Time: 10 minutes
Cooking time: 30 minutes
Servings: 3
Ingredients:

- 8 low carb tortilla shells
- 6 eggs
- 1 cup water
- 3 tablespoon butter
- 1 ½ cups grated cheddar cheese
- 1 ½ cups grated Swiss cheese
- 5 bacon slices
- 1 medium onion, thinly sliced
- 1 tablespoon chopped parsley

Directions

1. Bring the eggs to a boil in water over medium heat for 10 minutes. Transfer the eggs to an ice water bath, peel the shells, and chop them; set aside.
2. Meanwhile, as the eggs cook, fry the bacon in a skillet over medium heat for 4 minutes until crispy. Remove and chop. Plate and set aside too.
3. Fetch out 2/3 of the bacon fat and sauté the onions in the remaining grease over medium heat for 2 minutes; set aside. Melt 1 tablespoon of butter in a skillet over medium heat.
4. Lay one tortilla in a skillet; sprinkle with some Swiss cheese. Add some chopped eggs and bacon over the cheese, top with onion, and sprinkle with some cheddar cheese. Cover with another tortilla shell. Cook for 45 seconds, then carefully flip the quesadilla, and cook the other side too for 45 seconds. Remove to a plate and repeat the cooking process using the remaining tortilla shells.
5. Garnish with parsley and serve warm.

Nutrition:

Kcal 449,
Fat 48.7g,
Net Carbs 6.8g,
Protein 29.1g

Bacon and Cheese Frittata

Preparation Time: 10 minutes
Cooking time: 20 minutes
Servings: 3
Ingredients:

- 10 slices bacon
- 10 fresh eggs
- 3 tablespoon butter, melted
- ½ cup almond milk
- Salt and black pepper to taste
- 1 ½ cups cheddar cheese, shredded
- ¼ cup chopped green onions

Directions:

1. Preheat the oven to 400ºF and grease a baking dish with cooking spray. Cook the bacon in a skillet over medium heat for 6 minutes. Once crispy, remove from the skillet to paper towels and discard grease. Chop into small pieces. Whisk the eggs, butter, milk, salt, and black pepper. Mix in the bacon and pour the mixture into the baking dish.
2. Sprinkle with cheddar cheese and green onions, and bake in the oven for 10 minutes or until the eggs are thoroughly cooked. Remove and cool the frittata for 3 minutes, slice into wedges, and serve warm with a dollop of Greek yogurt.

Nutrition:
Kcal 325,
Fat 28g,
Net Carbs 2g,
Protein 15g

Spicy Egg Muffins with Bacon & Cheese

Preparation Time: 10 minutes
Cooking time: 20 minutes
Servings: 3
Ingredients:

- 12 eggs
- ¼ cup coconut milk
- Salt and black pepper to taste
- 1 cup grated cheddar cheese
- 12 slices bacon
- 4 jalapeño peppers, seeded and minced

Directions:

1. Preheat oven to 370ºF.
2. Crack the eggs into a bowl and whisk with coconut milk until combined. Season with salt and pepper, and evenly stir in the cheddar cheese.
3. Line each hole of a muffin tin with a slice of bacon and fill each with the egg mixture two-thirds way up. Top with the jalapeno peppers and bake in the oven for 18 to 20 minutes or until puffed and golden. Remove, allow cooling for a few minutes, and serve with arugula salad.

Nutrition:
Kcal 302,
Fat 23.7g,
Net Carbs 3.2g,
Protein 20g

Ham & Egg Broccoli Bake

Preparation Time: 10 minutes
Cooking time: 25 minutes
Servings: 3
Ingredients:

- 2 heads broccoli, cut into small florets
- 2 red bell peppers, seeded and chopped
- ¼ cup chopped ham
- 2 teaspoon ghee
- 1 teaspoon dried oregano + extra to garnish
- Salt and black pepper to taste
- 8 fresh eggs

Directions

1. Preheat oven to 425ºF.
2. Melt the ghee in a frying pan over medium heat; brown the ham, stirring frequently, about 3 minutes.
3. Arrange the broccoli, bell peppers, and ham on a foil-lined baking sheet in a single layer, toss to combine; season with salt, oregano, and black pepper. Bake for 10 minutes until the vegetables have softened.
4. Remove, create eight indentations with a spoon, and crack an egg into each. Return to the oven and continue to bake for an additional 5 to 7 minutes until the egg whites are firm.
5. Season with salt, black pepper, and extra oregano, share the bake into four plates and serve with strawberry lemonade (optional).

Nutrition:
Kcal 344,
Fat 28g,
Net Carbs 4.2g,
Protein 11g

Hot Buffalo wings

Preparation Time: 10 minutes
Cooking Time: 47 minutes
Servings: 3
Ingredients:

- Hot sauce ¼ cup
- Coconut oil 4 tablespoons, plus more for rubbing on the wings
- Chicken wings 12 (fresh or frozen)
- Garlic 1 clove, minced
- Salt ¼ teaspoon
- Paprika ¼ teaspoon
- Cayenne pepper ¼ teaspoon
- Ground black pepper 1 dash

Directions:

1. Preheat your oven to 400 degrees F (200 degrees C).
2. Evenly spread chicken wings on a wire rack placed on a baking dish (it will save wings to become soggy on the bottom).
3. Rub each chicken wing with olive oil and season with salt and pepper, then bake for 45 minutes, or until crispy.

4. Meanwhile, in a saucepan combine coconut oil and garlic and cook over medium heat for 1 minute, or until fragrant.
5. Remove from heat and stir in hot sauce, salt, paprika, cayenne pepper and black pepper.
6. Remove wings from the oven and transfer to a large bowl.
7. Pour hot sauce mixture over wings and toss until each wing is coated with the sauce.
8. Serve immediately.

Nutrition:
Calories: 391
Carbohydrates: 1 g
Fats: 33 g
Protein: 31 g

Turkey Meatballs

Preparation Time: 30 minutes
Cooking Time: 0 minutes
Servings: 4
Ingredients:

- 255g turkey sausage
- 2 tablespoons of extra virgin olive oil
- One can of 425g chickpeas, rinsed and drained...
- 1/2 medium onion, chopped, 2/3 cup
- 2 cloves of garlic, finely chopped
- 1 teaspoon of cumin
- 1/2 cup flour
- 1/2 teaspoon instant yeast for desserts
- Salt and ground black pepper
- 1 cup of Greek yogurt
- 2 tablespoons of lime juice
- 2 radicchio hearts, chopped
- Hot sauce

Directions:

1. Preheat the oven to 200°C.
2. In a processor, blend the chickpeas, onion, garlic, cumin, 1 teaspoon salt and 1/2 teaspoon pepper until all the ingredients are finely chopped. Add the flour, baking powder and blend to make everything mix well. Transfer to a medium bowl and add the sausage, stirring together with your hands. Cover and refrigerate for 30 minutes.
3. Once cold, take the mixture in spoonful, forming 1-inch balls with wet hands. Heat the olive oil in a pan over medium heat. In two groups, put the falafel in the pan and cook until slightly brown, about a minute and a half per side. Transfer to a baking tray and bake in the oven until well cooked, for about 10 minutes.

4. Mix together the yogurt, lime juice, 1/2 teaspoon salt and 1/4 teaspoon pepper. Divide the lettuce into 4 plates, season with some yogurt sauce.

Nutrition:
Calories 189
Fat 5
Protein 77
Sugar 3

Chicken in Sweet and Sour Sauce with Corn Salad

Preparation Time: 10 minutes
Cooking Time: 15 minutes
Servings: 4
Ingredients:

- 2 cups plus 2 tablespoons of unflavored low-fat yoghurt
- 2 cups of frozen mango chunks
- 3 tablespoons of honey
- ¼ cup plus 1 tablespoon apple cider vinegar
- ¼ cup sultana
- 2 tablespoons of olive oil, plus an amount to be brushed
- ¼ teaspoon of cayenne pepper
- 5 dried tomatoes (not in oil)
- 2 small cloves of garlic, finely chopped
- 4 cobs, peeled
- 8 peeled and boned chicken legs, peeled (about 700g)
- Halls
- 6 cups of mixed salad
- 2 medium carrots, finely sliced

Directions:

1. For the smoothie: in a blender, mix 2 cups of yogurt, 2 cups of ice, 1 cup of mango and all the honey until the mixture becomes completely smooth. Divide into 4 glasses and refrigerate until ready to use. Rinse the blender.
2. Preheat the grill to medium-high heat. Mix the remaining cup of mango, ¼ cup water, ¼ cup vinegar, sultanas, olive oil, cayenne pepper, tomatoes and garlic in a microwave bowl. Cover with a piece of clear film and cook in the microwave until the tomatoes become soft, for about 3 minutes. Leave to cool slightly and pass in a blender. Transfer to a small bowl. Leave 2 tablespoons aside to garnish, turn the chicken into the remaining mixture.

3. Put the corn on the grill, cover and bake, turning it over if necessary, until it is burnt, about 10 minutes. Remove and keep warm.

4. Brush the grill over medium heat and brush the grills with a little oil. Turn the chicken legs into half the remaining sauce and ½ teaspoon of salt. Put on the grill and cook until the cooking marks appear and the internal temperature reaches 75°C on an instantaneous thermometer, 8 to 10 minutes per side. Bart and sprinkle a few times with the remaining sauce while cooking.

5. While the chicken is cooking, beat the remaining 2 tablespoons of yogurt, the 2 tablespoons of sauce set aside, the remaining spoonful of vinegar, 1 tablespoon of water and ¼ teaspoon of salt in a large bowl. Mix the mixed salad with the carrots. Divide chicken, corn and salad into 4 serving dishes. Garnish the salad with the dressing set aside. Serve each plate with a mango smoothie.

Nutrition:
Calories 346
Protein 56
Fat 45

Chinese Chicken Salad

Preparation Time: 15 minutes
Cooking Time: 30 minutes
Servings: 4
Ingredients:

- For the chicken salad:
- 4 divided chicken breasts with skin and bones
- Olive oil of excellent quality
- Salt and freshly ground black pepper
- 500 g asparagus, with the ends removed and cut into three parts diagonally
- 1 red pepper, peeled
- Chinese condiment, recipe to follow
- 2 spring onions (both the white and the green part), sliced diagonally
- 1 tablespoon of white sesame seeds, toasted
- For Chinese dressing:
- 120 ml vegetable oil
- 60 ml of apple cider vinegar of excellent quality
- 60 ml soy sauce
- 1 ½ tablespoon of black sesame
- ½ tablespoon of honey
- 1 clove of garlic, minced

- ½ teaspoon of fresh peeled and grated ginger
- ½ tablespoon sesame seeds, toasted
- 60 g peanut butter
- 2 teaspoons of salt
- ½ teaspoons freshly ground black pepper

Directions:

1. For the chicken salad:
2. Heat the oven to 180°C (or 200°C for gas oven). Put the chicken breast on a baking tray and rub the skin with a little olive oil. Season freely with salt and pepper.
3. Brown for 35 to 40 minutes, until the chicken is freshly cooked. Let it cool down as long as it takes to handle it. Remove the meat from the bones, remove the skin and chop the chicken into medium-sized pieces.
4. Blanch the asparagus in a pot of salted water for 3-5 minutes until tender. Soak them in water with ice to stop cooking. Drain them. Cut the peppers into strips the same size as the asparagus. In a large bowl, mix the chopped chicken, asparagus and peppers.
5. Spread the Chinese dressing on chicken and vegetables. Add the spring onions and sesame seeds, and season to taste. Serve cold or at room temperature.
6. For Chinese dressing:
7. Mix all ingredients and set aside until use.

Nutrition:
Calories 222
Protein 28
Fat 10
Sugar 6

Chicken Salad

Preparation Time: 15 minutes
Cooking Time: 25 minutes
Servings: 4
Ingredients:

- For the Buffalo chicken salad:
- 2 chicken breasts (225 g) peeled, boned, cut in half
- 2 tablespoons of hot cayenne pepper sauce (or another type of hot sauce), plus an addition depending on taste
- 2 tablespoons of olive oil
- 2 romaine lettuce heart, cut into 2 cm strips
- 4 celery stalks, finely sliced
- 2 carrots, roughly grated
- 2 fresh onions, only the green part, sliced
- 125 ml of blue cheese dressing, recipe to follow
- For the seasoning of blue cheese
- 2 tablespoons mayonnaise
- 70 ml of partially skimmed buttermilk
- 70 ml low-fat white yoghurt
- 1 tablespoon of wine vinegar
- ½ teaspoon of sugar
- 35 g of chopped blue cheese
- Salt and freshly ground black pepper

Directions:

1. For the Buffalo chicken salad:
2. Preheat the grid.
3. Place the chicken between 2 sheets of baking paper and beat it with a meat tenderizer so that it is about 2 cm thick, then cut the chicken sideways creating 1 cm strips.

4. In a large bowl, add the hot sauce and oil, add the chicken and turn it over until it is well soaked. Place the chicken on a baking tray and grill until well cooked, about 4-6 minutes, turning it once.

5. In a large bowl, add the lettuce, celery, grated carrots and fresh onions. Add the seasoning of blue cheese. Distribute the vegetables in 4 plates and arrange the chicken on each of the dishes. Serve with hot sauce on the side.

6. For the blue cheese dressing:

7. Cover a small bowl with absorbent paper folded in four. Spread the yoghurt on the paper and put it in the fridge for 20 minutes to drain and firm it.

8. In a medium bowl, beat the buttermilk and firm yogurt with mayonnaise until well blended. Add the vinegar and sugar and keep beating until well blended. Add the blue cheese and season with salt and pepper to taste.

Nutrition:
321 calories
Fat 3
Fiber 5
Carbs 7
Protein 4

Avocado and Kale Eggs

Preparation Time: 10 minutes
Cooking time: 30 minutes
Servings: 3
Ingredients:

- 1 teaspoon ghee
- 1 red onion, sliced
- 4 oz. chorizo, sliced into thin rounds
- 1 cup chopped kale
- 1 ripe avocado, pitted, peeled, chopped
- 4 eggs
- Salt and black pepper to season

Directions:

1. Preheat oven to 370ºF.
2. Melt ghee in a cast iron pan over medium heat and sauté the onion for 2 minutes. Add the chorizo and cook for 2 minutes more, flipping once.
3. Introduce the kale in batches with a splash of water to wilt, season lightly with salt, stir and cook for 3 minutes. Mix in the avocado and turn the heat off.
4. Create four holes in the mixture, crack the eggs into each hole, sprinkle with salt and black pepper, and slide the pan into the preheated oven to bake for 6 minutes until the egg whites are set or firm and yolks still runny. Season to taste with salt and pepper, and serve right away with low carb toasts.

Nutrition:
Kcal 274,
Fat 23g,
Net Carbs 4g,
Protein 13g

Tofu Meat and Salad

Preparation Time: 15 minutes
Cooking Time: 20 minutes
Servings: 3
Ingredients:

- 1 tablespoon of garlic sauce and chili in a bottle
- 1 1/2 tablespoon sesame oil
- 3 tablespoons of low-sodium soy sauce
- 60 ml hoisin sauce
- 2 tablespoons rice vinegar
- 2 tablespoons of sherry or Chinese cooking wine
- 225 g of extra-solid tofu
- 2 teaspoons of rapeseed oil
- 2 tablespoons of finely chopped fresh ginger
- 4 spring onions, with the green part chopped and set aside, in thin slices
- 225 g of minced lean beef (90% or more lean)
- 25 g of diced Chinese water chestnuts
- 1 large head of cappuccino lettuce, with the leaves separated, but without the outer ones
- 1 red pepper, diced

Directions:

- In a bowl, mix together the garlic and chili sauce, sesame oil, soy sauce, hoisin sauce, vinegar and sherry.
- Cut the tofu into 1 cm thick slices and place them on a kitchen towel. Use the cloth to dab the tofu well to remove as much water as possible. Should take a couple of minutes and about three dish towels. Chop the dry tofu well and set aside.
- Heat the oil in a wok or in a very large pan and medium flame. Add the ginger and the white part of the spring onions and cook until the spring onions become translucent and the ginger fragrant, for about 2-3 minutes. Add the beef and tofu and cook, stirring, until the meat becomes dull and freshly cooked, for about 4-5 minutes. Add the sauce set aside. Reduce the

flame and simmer slowly, stirring, for another 3-4 minutes. Add the chestnuts and mix well to incorporate.

• Fill each lettuce leaf with stuffing. Serve by decorating with the green part of the spring onions, red pepper and peanuts.

Nutrition:
Calories 122
Fat 2
Protein 66

Asparagus and Pistachios Vinaigrette

Preparation Time: 10 minutes
Cooking Time: 5minutes
Servings: 2
Ingredients:

- Two 455g bunches of large asparagus, without the tip
- 1 tablespoon of olive oil
- Salt and freshly ground black pepper
- 6 tablespoons of sliced pistachios blanched and boiled
- 1 1/2 tablespoon lemon juice
- 1/4 teaspoon of sugar
- 1 1/2 teaspoon lemon zest

Directions:

1. Preheat the oven to 220°C. Put the grill in the top third of the oven. Place the asparagus on a baking tray covered with baking paper. Sprinkle with olive oil and season with a little salt and pepper. Bake for 15 minutes, until soft.
2. Meanwhile, blend 5 tablespoons of almonds, lemon juice, sugar and 6 tablespoons of water for 1 minute until smooth. Taste and regulate salt. Pour the sauce on a plate and put the spinach on the sauce. Decorate with peel and the remaining spoon of pistachios

Nutrition:
Calories 560
Fat 5
Fiber 2
Carbs 3
Protein 9

Chili Cauliflower Mix

Preparation Time: 10 minutes
Cooking Time: 35 minutes
Servings: 4
Ingredients:

- 2 tablespoons sweet chili sauce
- 3 tablespoons olive oil
- 3 garlic cloves, minced
- Juice of 1 lime
- 1 cauliflower head, florets separated
- 1 teaspoon cilantro, chopped
- A pinch of salt and black pepper

Directions:

1. In a bowl, the chili sauce with the oil, garlic, lime juice, salt, pepper, cilantro and the cauliflower, toss well, spread on a lined baking sheet, introduce in the oven and cook at 425 degrees F for 35 minutes.
2. Divide the cauliflower between plates and serve as a side dish.

Nutrition:
Calories: 271
Fat: 4
Fiber: 7,
Carbohydrates: 11
Protein: 7

Mozzarella Brussels Sprouts

Preparation Time: 10 minutes
Cooking Time: 30 minutes
Servings: 6
Ingredients:

- 2 tablespoons olive oil
- 2 pounds Brussels sprouts
- 2 garlic cloves, minced
- 1 teaspoon thyme, chopped
- A pinch of salt and black pepper
- 1 cup mozzarella, shredded
- ¼ cup parmesan, grated
- 1 tablespoon parsley, chopped

Directions:

1. Put some water in a pot, bring to a boil over medium-high heat, add sprouts, cook them for 10 minutes, transfer them to a bowl filled with ice water, cool them down and drain them well.
2. In a bowl, combine the Brussels sprouts with salt, pepper, oil, garlic and thyme, toss and smash them a bit.
3. Spread smashed Brussels sprouts on a lined baking sheet, sprinkle mozzarella and parmesan on top, introduce in the oven and bake them at 425 degrees F for 20 minutes.
4. Sprinkle parsley on top, divide between plates and serve as a side dish.

Nutrition:
Calories: 288
Fat: 4
Fiber: 6
Carbohydrates: 13
Protein: 6

Mozzarella Broccoli Mix

Preparation Time: 10 minutes
Cooking Time: 15 minutes
Servings: 4
Ingredients:

- 2 tablespoons olive oil
- 1 broccoli head, florets separated
- 2 garlic cloves, minced
- ½ cup mozzarella, shredded
- ¼ cup parmesan, grated
- ½ cup coconut cream
- 1 tablespoon parsley, chopped

Directions:

1. Heat up a pan with the oil over medium-high heat add broccoli, salt, pepper and garlic, stir and cook for 6 minutes.
2. Add parmesan, mozzarella and cream, toss, introduce the pan in the oven and cook at 375 degrees F for 10 minutes.
3. Add parsley, toss, divide between plates and serve as a side dish.

Nutrition:
Calories: 261
Fat: 4
Fiber: 4
Carbohydrates: 13
Protein: 8

Parsley Bacon Brussels Sprouts

Preparation Time: 10 minutes
Cooking Time: 20 minutes
Servings: 6
Ingredients:

- 1-pound Brussels sprouts, halved
- A pinch of salt and black pepper
- 7 bacon slices, chopped
- 1 yellow onion, chopped
- 2 tablespoons stevia
- 2 tablespoons olive oil
- 1 tablespoon parsley, chopped
- 2 teaspoons sweet paprika

Directions:

1. Heat up a pan with the oil over medium-high heat, add the onion, stir and sauté for 4-5 minutes.
2. Add the bacon, stir and cook for 3 minutes more.
3. Add the sprouts, salt, pepper, stevia, paprika and parsley, toss, cook for 10 minutes more, divide between plates and serve as a side dish.

Nutrition:
Calories: 261
Fat: 4
Fiber: 8
Carbohydrates: 12
Protein: 8

Mediterranean Side Salad

Preparation Time: 10 minutes
Cooking Time: 0 minutes
Servings: 4
Ingredients:

- 1-pint cherry tomatoes, halved
- 1 cup kalamata olives, pitted and sliced
- 1 cucumber, sliced
- ½ red onion, sliced
- 1 cup feta cheese, crumbled
- Juice of ½ lemon
- 2 tablespoons red vinegar
- A pinch of salt and black pepper
- 1 teaspoon oregano, dried
- ¼ cup olive oil

Directions:

1. In a salad bowl, combine the tomatoes with the olives, cucumber and onion.
2. In a separate bowl, combine the lemon juice with the vinegar, salt, pepper, oregano and oil and whisk well.
3. Pour this over your salad, toss, sprinkle cheese at the end and serve as a side dish.

Nutrition:
Calories: 200
Fat: 3
Fiber: 6
Carbohydrates: 12
Protein: 8

Mozzarella and Artichoke Mix

Preparation Time: 10 minutes
Cooking Time: 10 minutes
Servings: 4
Ingredients:

- 14 ounces canned artichoke hearts, drained
- A pinch of salt and black pepper
- 2 cups baby spinach
- 2 tablespoons parsley, chopped
- 1 cup mozzarella, shredded
- Juice of 1 lemon
- 1 and ¾ cup coconut milk
- ½ cup chicken stock
- 2 garlic cloves, minced
- 3 tablespoons ghee, melted
- A pinch of red pepper flakes

Directions:

1. Heat up a pan with the ghee over medium-high heat, add the garlic, stir and cook for 2 minutes.
2. Add lemon juice, coconut milk, stock, artichokes, salt and pepper, stir and cook for 5 minutes.
3. Add spinach, pepper flakes and mozzarella, toss, cook for 3 minutes more, and divide between plates, sprinkle parsley on top and serve as a side dish.

Nutrition:
Calories: 277
Fat: 3
Fiber: 6
Carbohydrates: 12

Protein: 8

Roasted Brussels Sprouts

Preparation Time: 10 minutes
Cooking Time: 25 minutes
Servings: 4
Ingredients:

- 1-pound Brussels sprouts, halved
- 2 tablespoons olive oil
- A pinch of salt and black pepper

Directions:

1. Spread the sprouts on a lined baking sheet, add the oil, salt and pepper, toss, introduce in the oven and bake at 425 degrees F for 25 minutes.
2. Divide between plates and serve as a side dish.

Nutrition:
Calories: 200
Fat: 2
Fiber: 6
Carbohydrates: 11
Protein: 8

Rosemary Veggie Mix

Preparation Time: 10 minutes
Cooking Time: 20 minutes
Servings: 4
Ingredients:

- 1-pound Brussels sprouts, halved
- 2 tablespoons olive oil
- 1 teaspoon rosemary, chopped
- 1 tablespoon balsamic vinegar
- 1 teaspoon thyme, chopped
- ½ cup cranberries, dried

Directions:

1. Spread the sprouts on a lined baking sheet, add rosemary, vinegar, oil and thyme, toss, introduce in the oven and cook at 400 degrees F for 20 minutes.
2. Divide between plates, sprinkle cranberries on top and serve as a side dish.

Nutrition:
Calories: 199
Fat: 3
Fiber: 5
Carbohydrates: 12
Protein: 7

Citric Cauliflower Rice

Preparation Time: 10 minutes
Cooking Time: 15 minutes
Servings: 4
Ingredients:

- 1 tablespoon ghee, melted
- Juice of 2 limes
- A pinch of salt and black pepper
- 1 cup cauliflower rice
- 1 and ½ cups veggie stock
- 1 tablespoon cilantro, chopped

Directions:

1. Heat up a pan with the ghee over medium-high heat, add the cauliflower rice, stir and cook for 5 minutes.
2. Add lime juice, salt, pepper and stock, stir, bring to a simmer and cook for 10 minutes.
3. Add cilantro, toss, divide between plates and serve as a side dish.

Nutrition:
Calories: 200
Fat: 3
Fiber: 6
Carbohydrates: 9
Protein: 6

Zoodles Side Dish

Preparation Time: 10 minutes
Cooking Time: 0 minutes
Servings: 4
Ingredients:

- 4 zucchinis, cut with a spiralizer
- 2 tablespoons olive oil
- A pinch of salt and black pepper
- 1 cup mozzarella, shredded
- 2 cups cherry tomatoes, halved
- ¼ cup basil, torn
- 2 tablespoons balsamic vinegar

Directions:

1. In a bowl, combine the zucchini noodles with salt, pepper and the oil, toss and leave aside for 10 minutes.
2. Add mozzarella, tomatoes, basil and vinegar, toss, divide between plates and serve as a side dish.

Nutrition:
Calories: 188
Fat: 6
Fiber: 8
Carbohydrates: 8
Protein: 6

Coconut Cauliflower Mash

Preparation Time: 10 minutes
Cooking Time: 10 minutes
Servings: 6
Ingredients:

- 2 cauliflower heads, florets separated
- 1/3 cup coconut cream
- 1/3 cup coconut milk
- 1 tablespoon chives, chopped
- A pinch of salt and black pepper

Directions:

1. Put some water in a pot, bring to a boil over medium-high heat, add cauliflower florets, cook them for 10 minutes, drain them well, mash using a potato masher and stir.
2. Add the cream, the coconut milk, salt, pepper and chives, stir well, divide between plates and serve as a side dish.

Nutrition:
Calories: 200
Fat: 3
Fiber: 3
Carbohydrates: 12
Protein: 5

Parmesan Brussels Sprouts

Preparation Time: 10 minutes
Cooking Time: 30 minutes
Servings: 4
Ingredients:

- 1-pound Brussels sprouts, halved
- 1 teaspoon oregano, dried
- 1 tablespoon olive oil
- 3 garlic cloves, minced
- ½ teaspoon hot paprika
- A pinch of salt and black pepper
- 2 tablespoons keto ranch dressing
- 1 tablespoon parmesan, grated

Directions:

1. Spread the sprouts on a lined baking sheet, add oregano, oil, garlic, paprika, salt and pepper, toss, bake them in the oven at 425 degrees F for 30 minutes, add parmesan and keto ranch dressing, toss well, divide between plates and serve as a side dish.

Nutrition:
Calories: 222
Fat: 4
Fiber: 6
Carbohydrates: 12
Protein: 8

Fried Cauliflower Rice

Preparation Time: 10 minutes
Cooking Time: 15 minutes
Servings: 4
Ingredients:

- 1 tablespoon ghee, melted
- 1 small yellow onion, chopped
- 2 hot dogs, sliced
- 1 tablespoon avocado oil
- 1 garlic clove, minced
- 2 and ½ cups cauliflower rice, steamed
- 2 eggs, whisked
- 2 tablespoons coconut amino
- 2 scallions, sliced

Directions:

1. Heat up a pan with the ghee over medium-high heat, add onion, garlic and hot dogs, stir and cook for 5 minutes.
2. Add cauliflower rice and avocado oil, stir and cook for 5 minutes more.
3. Add the eggs, toss everything, and cook for 5 more minutes until the eggs are scrambled, add the amino and the scallions, toss, divide between plates and serve as a side dish.

Nutrition:
Calories: 200
Fat: 3
Fiber: 6
Carbohydrates: 12
Protein: 8

Cheesy Asparagus Dish

Preparation Time: 10 minutes
Cooking Time: 30 minutes
Servings: 6
Ingredients:

- 3 garlic cloves, minced
- ¾ cup coconut cream
- 2 pounds asparagus, trimmed
- 1 cup parmesan, grated
- A pinch of salt and black pepper
- 1 cup mozzarella, shredded

Directions:

1. In a baking dish, combine the asparagus with the garlic, cream, salt, pepper, mozzarella and top with the parmesan, introduce in the oven and bake at 400 degrees F for 30 minutes.
2. Divide between plates and serve as a side dish.

Nutrition:
Calories: 200
Fat: 3
Fiber: 6
Carbohydrates: 12
Protein: 9

Roasted Cauliflower with Prosciutto, Capers, and Almonds.

Preparation Time: 10 minutes
Cooking Time: 25 minutes
Servings: 2
Ingredients:

- 12 ounces cauliflower florets (I get precut florets at Trader Joe's)
- 2 tablespoons leftover bacon grease, or olive oil
- Pink Himalayan salt
- Freshly ground black pepper
- 2 ounces sliced prosciutto, torn into small pieces
- ¼ cup slivered almonds
- 2 tablespoons capers
- 2 tablespoons grated Parmesan cheese

Directions:

1. Preheat the oven to 400 degrees F. Line a baking pan with a silicone baking mat or parchment paper.
2. Put the cauliflower florets in the prepared baking pan with the bacon grease, and season with pink Himalayan salt and pepper. Or if you are using olive oil instead, drizzle the cauliflower with olive oil and season with pink Himalayan salt and pepper.
3. Roast the cauliflower for 15 minutes.
4. Stir the cauliflower so all sides are coated with the bacon grease.
5. Distribute the prosciutto pieces in the pan. Then add the slivered almonds and capers. Stir to combine. Sprinkle the Parmesan cheese on top, and roast for 10 minutes more.
6. Divide between two plates, using a slotted spoon so you don't get excess grease in the plates, and serve.

Nutrition:
Calories: 288

Fat: 24g
Carbohydrates: 7
Fiber: 3
Protein: 14

Keto Jalapeno Poppers

Preparation Time: 10 minutes
Cooking Time: 20 minutes
Serving: 16
Ingredients

- 8 oz. cream cheese
- 1/2 cup shredded sharp cheddar cheese
- 1 tsp pink himalayan salt
- 1/2 tsp black pepper
- 8 jalapenos, halved, de-seeded
- 8 slices of bacon, cut in half

Directions:

1. Preheat stove to 375 degrees and line heating sheet with material paper.
2. Spot bacon cuts on paper towel-lined plate and microwave for 3 minutes. Put aside to somewhat cool.
3. In a medium bowl, include cream cheddar, destroyed sharp cheddar, salt, and pepper and microwave for 15 seconds. Mix together
4. Cautiously scoop cream cheddar blend into a plastic baggie

5. Wrap bacon cuts around jalapenos and stick with a toothpick.

6. Spot jalapenos on arranged heating sheet and prepare for 15 minutes.

7. Increment broiler warmth to cook and sear for 2-3 minutes, watching to guarantee cream cheddar doesn't consume.

8. Remove from broiler and permit cooling marginally before eating.

Nutrition
Calories 79
Fat 6.6g,
Carbs 2.1g,
Protein 8g

Barbecue Fat Balls

Preparation Time: 5 minutes
Cooking Time: 0 minutes
Serving: 6
Ingredients

- 4 ounces cream cheese
- 4 tbsp. bacon fat
- ½ tsp smoke flavor
- 2 drops stevia
- 1/8 tsp apple cider vinegar
- 1 tbsp. sweet smoked chili powder

Directions:

1. In a food processor, process all ingredients except chili powder until they form a smooth cream.
2. Scrap mixture and transfer into a small bowl, then refrigerate for 2 hours.
3. Form into 6 balls.
4. Sprinkle balls with chili powder, roll to coat well.
5. Serve.

Nutrition
Calories 146
Fat 14g
Carbs 1.5g
Protein 1.3g

Bacon-Wrapped Scallops

Preparation Time: 10 minutes
    Cooking Time: 15 minute
    Serving: 4
    Ingredients

- 16 sea scallops
- 8 slices bacon
- 16 toothpicks
- olive oil for drizzling
- black pepper and kosher salt to taste

Directions:

1. Preheat broiler to 425°F.
2. Line a heating sheet with material paper. Put in a safe spot.
3. Envelop one scallop by using a half-reduce of bacon and comfortable with a toothpick.
4. Shower olive oil over every scallop and season with pepper and valid salt.
5. Orchestrate scallops in a solitary layer on a readied preparing sheet, giving every scallop some space to permit the bacon to clean.
6. Heat 12 to 15mins until scallop is sensitive and bacon is cooked through. Serve hot.

Nutrition
Calories 224
Fat 17g,
Carbs 2g, Protein 12g

Low Carb Tortilla Pork Rind Wraps

Preparation Time: 10 minutes
Cooking Time: 30 minutes
Serving: 8 wraps
Ingredients

- 4 large eggs
- 3 ounces pork rinds
- ½ tsp garlic powder
- ¼ tsp ground cumin
- ¼ to ½ cup water
- avocado oil or coconut oil

Directions:

1. In a powerful blender or nourishment processor, consolidate the eggs, pork skins, garlic powder, and cumin. Mix until smooth and very much joined. Include 1/4 cup of the water and mix once more. On the off chance that the blend is extremely thick, keep on including water until it is the consistency of hotcake hitter.
2. Warmth a sparse 1/2 teaspoon of oil in an 8-inch nonstick skillet over medium-low warmth, include around 3 tablespoons of the hitter and utilize an elastic spatula to spread it meagerly over the base of the dish, nearly to the edges.

3. Cook for about a moment, until the base is starting to dark-colored.

4. Rehash with the rest of the player, adding oil to the skillet just as essential

5. Add more water to the player as required; it will thicken as it sits.

Nutrition
Calories 194,
Fat 5.6g,
Carbs 5.4g,
Protein 9.7g

Avocado Chicken Salad

Preparation Time: 15 minutes
Cooking Time: 20 minutes
Serving: 3
Ingredients

- 3 avocados
- 1 lb. chicken (cooked in any way from this book)
- 1 medium tomato
- 1 onion
- 4 limes
- sea salt and fresh ground black pepper

Directions:

1. In an enormous bowl pound the avocados until smooth.
2. Include the chicken, onions, tomatoes, lime squeeze, salt, and pepper.
3. Blend well.

Nutrition
Calories 465,
Fat 38g,

Carbs 6.7g, Protein 55g

Paleo-Italian Carpaccio

Preparation Time: 1hour 30 minutes
Cooking Time: 1 hour
Serving: *4*
Ingredients

- 8 ounces of grass-fed, grass-finished filet mignon
- 1 bunch fresh organic Arugula
- 4 tsp truffle infused extra virgin olive oil
- 1 tsp unrefined sea salt
- freshly ground black pepper to taste

Directions:

1. Spot the meat in the cooler for around 2 hours. This will make it firm enough to cut with a sharp gourmet specialist's blade or with a meat slicer.
2. Cut meagerly and isolate the individual cuts laying them on 4 individual plates.
3. Organize the arugula over the meat, separating it similarly
4. Shower the oil on the plates, at that point sprinkle with salt and pepper
5. In the event that you are utilizing cheddar, mastermind the shaved parmesan on top
6. You can include extra naturally ground dark pepper to decorate the top.

7. Plates can be chilled in the icebox for 30 minutes before serving.

Nutrition
Calories 437, Fat 28g, Carbs 4g, Protein 31g

Meat-Lover Pizza Cups

Preparation Time: 15 minutes
Cooking Time: 11 minutes
Serving: 12
Ingredients

- 12 deli ham slices
- 1 lb. bulk Italian sausages
- 12 tbsp. sugar-free pizza sauce
- 3 cups grated mozzarella cheese
- 24 pepperoni slices
- 1 cup cooked and crumbled bacon

Directions:

1. Preheat broiler to 375 F. Fry Italian frankfurters in a skillet, depleting abundance oil.
2. Line 12-cup biscuit tin with ham cuts. Italian sausages, ham slices, pizza sauce, mozzarella cheese, pepperoni cuts, and bacon disintegrate between each cup, in a specific order.
3. Heat at 375 F for 10 minutes, cook for 1 moment until cheese air pockets and tans and the edges of the meat ingredients look firm.

4. Remove pizza cups from biscuit tin and set on paper towels to keep the bottoms from getting wet.
5. Serve.

Nutrition
Calories 165, Fat 14g, Carbs 6.1g, Protein 2g

Bacon Onion Butter

Preparation Time: 15 minutes
Cooking Time: 35 minutes
Serving: 6
Ingredients

- 9 tbsp. butter
- 4 strips bacon sliced into small strips
- 90 grams onion
- 2 tsp spicy brown mustard
- 1/2 tsp black pepper

Directions:

1. Dissolve 1 tablespoon margarine in a skillet on medium warmth and include bacon pieces.
2. When the bacon fat is beginning to cook include diced onion and fry until onion and bacon are fresh yet not overcooked.
3. Put aside bacon/onion blend in a bowl and cool to room temp.
4. Include mellowed margarine, 8 tablespoons, to an enormous blending bowl.
5. Include bacon and onions, yellow mustard, and pepper.
6. Cream together ingredients or utilize an electric blender.
7. Spoon into a smaller than normal biscuit tin, place in cooler until margarine is strong again.

Nutrition
Calories 830, Fat 117g, Carbs 7.0g, Protein 15g

Caesar Egg Salad Lettuce Wraps

Preparation Time: 10 minutes
Cooking Time: 15 minutes
Serving: 4
Ingredients

- 6 large hard-boiled eggs
- 3 tbsp. creamy Caesar dressing
- 3 tbsp. mayonnaise
- 1/2 cup Parmesan cheese
- cracked black pepper
- 4 large romaine lettuce leaves

Directions:

1. In a blending bowl, join hacked eggs, velvety Caesar dressing, mayonnaise, and 1/4 cup Parmesan cheddar and broke dark pepper.
2. Spoon blend onto romaine leaves and top with residual Parmesan cheddar.

Nutrition
Calories 254, Fat 22g, Carbs 2.7g, Protein 13.5g

Best Keto Popcorn Cheese Puffs

Preparation Time: 5 minutes

Cooking Time: 5 minutes

Servings: 4

Ingredients

• 4 ounces cheddar cheese sliced

Directions:

1. Cut the cheddar into little ¼ inch squares.
2. Prior to heating, this formula must be readied 24 hours in advance
3. Cover the pan with baking parchment.
4. Leave the cheddar to dry out for in any event 24 hours.
5. The following day preheat your stove to 200C/390F and heat the cheddar for 3-5 minutes until it is puffed up.
6. Leave to cool for 10 minutes before getting a charge out of.

Nutrition

Calories 114, Fat 9g, Carbs 2.2g, Protein 7g

Keto Bacon Wrapped Salmon with Pesto

Preparation Time: 5 minutes
Cooking Time: 15 minutes
Serving: 1
Ingredients

- 170g salmon fillet
- 1 slice streaky bacon
- 2 tbsp. pesto

Directions:

1. Spot the streaky bacon on a hacking board.
2. Spot the salmon filet over the bacon. Move up firmly and comfy with a wooden stick.
3. Spot 1-2 tbsp. pesto inside the center.
4. Spot in the skillet, unfold, and fry tenderly for 10 minutes until the salmon and bacon are cooked. There is not any compelling motive to show the keto bacon-wrapped salmon. At the factor when you prepare dinner it in the griddle with the top, on medium warm temperature, it'll permit the steam internal to cook dinner the salmon from above.
5. Then again, region the bacon-wrapped salmon on a covered making ready plate/sheet container within the stove at 180C/350F for 15mins

Nutrition
Calories 449, Fat 31g, Carbs 3g, Protein 38g

Deli Fat Bombs

Preparation Time: 5 minutes
Cooking Time: 0 minutes
Serving: 2
Ingredients

- 8 (1-ounce) slices sugar-free deli ham
- 4 ounces chive cream cheese
- 1 cup chopped baby spinach
- 1 medium red bell pepper, seeded and sliced

Directions:

1. Lay out each slice of ham flat. Spread 1 tbsp. cream cheese on each slice.
2. Put 2 tbsp. chopped spinach on top of the cream cheese on each slice.
3. Divide bell pepper into 8 portions and put the portions on top of spinach.
4. Roll up the ham and secure with a toothpick.
5. Serve.

Nutrition

Calories 399, Fat 25.9g, Carbs 6.7g, Protein 23.2g

Keto Low Carb Tortilla Chips

Preparation Time: 10 minutes
Cooking Time: 7 minutes
Servings: 8
Ingredients

- 2 cups mozzarella
- 3/4 cup almond flour
- 1/4 tsp onion, garlic and paprika
- 2 tbsp. psyllium husk Pinch salt

Directions:

1. Warmth you're stove to 350F.
2. Dissolve the mozzarella in the microwave. On the other hand, heat delicately in a non-stick pot.
3. Include the almond flour/ground almonds and psyllium husk in addition to the salt and flavors, if utilizing. Mix until consolidated, at that point ply until you have a smooth mixture.
4. Separate the batter into 2 balls and turn out between 2 sheets of preparing/material paper. Turn out as meagerly as could be expected under the circumstances! The more slender, the crispier your tortilla chips will turn out.

5. Cut into triangles and spread out on a sheet of preparing paper so the tortilla chips don't contact.

6. Prepare 6-8 minutes or until sautéed on the edges. Heating time will rely upon the thickness of your tortilla chips. I heated mine in 2 rounds, in addition to a third-round for the off-cuts.

Nutrition
Calories 143,
Fat 9.2g, Carbs 4.8g,
Protein 8.3g

21 Day Meal Plan

PlaRaspberries

Low-carb Snack List

1/4 cup: 16 calories, 0.20g fat, 3.67g carbs, 2g fiber, 0.37g protein 1/2 cup: 32 calories, 0.40g fat, 7.34g carbs, 4g fiber, 0.75g protein 1 cup: 64 calories, 0.80g fat, 14.69g carbs, 8g fiber, 1.48g protein Blueberries

1/4 cup: 21 calories, 0.12g fat, 5.25g carbs, 0.9g fiber, 0.27g protein

1/2 cup: 41 calories, 0.24g fat, 10.51g carbs, 1.7g fiber, 0.54g protein 1 cup: 83 calories, 0.48g fat, 21.01g carbs, 3.5g fiber, 1.07g protein Strawberries

1/4 cup: 12 calories, 0.11g fat, 2.92g carbs, 0.8g fiber, 0.25g protein 1/2 cup: 24 calories, 0.23g fat, 5.84g carbs, 1.5g fiber, 0.51g protein 1cup: 49 calories, 0.46g fat, 11.67g carbs, 3g fiber, 1.07g protein

Blackberries

1/4 cup: 15 calories, 0.18g fat, 3.46g carbs, 1.9g fiber, 0.5g protein 1/2 cup: 31 calories, 0.35g fat, 6.92g carbs, 3.8g fiber, 1g protein 1cup: 62 calories, 0.71g fat, 13.84g carbs, 7.6g fiber, 2g protein Nuts (Raw)

Almonds

1/4 cup: 160 calories, 14g fat, 6g carbs, 4g fiber, 6g protein

Cashews

1/4 cup: 160 calories, 12g fat, 8g carbs, 1g fiber, 5g protein Pecans

1/4 cup: 210 calories, 21g fat, 4g carbs, 2g fiber, 3g protein

Walnuts

1/4 cup: 190 calories, 18g fat, 4g carbs, 2g fiber, 4g protein Boiled Egg

1egg: 78 calories, 5.3g fat, 0.56g carbs, 0g fiber, 6.29g protein

Avocado

1/2 fruit: 161 calories, 14.73g fat, 8.57g carbs, 6.7g fiber, 2.01g protein Kalamata Olives

10 olives: 90 calories, 9g fat, 2g carbs, 2g fiber, 2g protein Almond Nut Butter

2 tbsp: 190 calories, 18g fat, 6g carbs, 3g fiber, 7g protein

Peeled Cucumber

1cup: 16 calories, 0.21g fat, 2.87g carbs, 2.8g fiber, 0.78g protein Celery Sticks

2 sticks: 15 calories, 0g fat, 4g carbs, 2g fiber, 1g protein

The following snack ideas depend on the brand or preparation method. Deviled Egg

Can of tuna

Cold meat –Leftover from a roast or deli meat like ham, salami, chicken, beef, etc.

Week 1 Menu

	Breakfast	Lunch	Dinner	Nutritional Info
Day 1	Avocado Bun Breakfast Burger	Avocado Cream & Zoodles	Chicken Cutlet and Cauli Rice	1765 calories 139.05g fat 20.75g net carbs 12.16g sugars 90.91g protein
Day 2	Breakfast Sausage, Eggs & Greens	Chicken Cutlet & Cauli Rice Leftovers	Shirataki Noodles Asian Salad	1374 calories 93g fat 19.79g net carbs 12.35g sugars 98.61g protein
Day 3	Breakfast Sausage & Eggs	BLT Lettuce Boats	Grilled Cod & Shrimps	1177calories 78.94g fat 15.74g net carbs 6.92g sugars 94.65g net carbs
Day 4	90 sec Sausage Egg Muffin	Grilled Cod & Shrimps Leftovers	Arugula Caesar Salad & Veggies	1316 calories 89g fat 19.75g net carbs 11.92g sugars 99.06g protein
Day 5	Breakfast Sausage& Poached Egg	Rosemary Chicken & Broccoli	Rosemary Pork Roast Leftovers Side Caesar Salad 3	1495 calories 111.31gfat 12.34g net carbs 7.29g sugars 101.2g protein
Day 6	Spinach & Breakfast Sausage Omelette	Rosemary Pork Roast Leftovers Side Caesar Salad 2	Broccoli, Bacon & Mushrooms	1313 calories 99.55g fat 13.02g net carbs 9.71g sugars 84.98g protein

Day 7 6	Spinach & Pork Omelette Leftovers	Zucchini Salad with Grilled Chicken Thigh	Rosemary Pork Roast Leftovers Side Caesar Salad 1	1509 calories 114.98g fat 15.62g net carbs 10.28g sugars 96.37g protein

Week 1 Grocery List

Baking
Baking Powder [1/2 tsp]
Blanched Almond Flour [7 tbsp]
Pork Rinds [40g]
Condiments
Anchovy Paste [10 ml]
Coconus Aminos [25 ml]
Fish Sauce [5 ml]
Lemon Juice [25 ml]
Mayonnaise [125 ml]
White Vinegar [20 ml]
Dairy
Almond Milk [45ml]
Eggs [19]
Meat
Bacon [5 slices]
Chicken Breast [1] {260g}skinless
Chicken Thighs [3] {200g} boneless
Ground Chicken [220g]
Ground Pork [220g]
Pork Roast Boneless [500g]
Prosciutto [60g]
Oil
Chili Oil [1/4 tsp](orcayenne pepper)
Frying Oil (Could be refined coconut oil, lard orbeef tallow)
Olive oil [215ml]
Refined Coconut Oil [15ml]
Sesame Oil [35ml]
Seafood & Fish
Cod Fillets [2] {300g}
Shrimps [200g]

Spices
Black Pepper
Cayenne Pepper
Celery Seed
Dashi Powder (Japanese Fish Broth Granule)
Garlic Powder
Himalayan Salt
Nutmeg
Onion Powder
Oregano
Paprika Powder
Parsley
Rosemary
Sage
Sesame Seeds
Thyme
Vegetables
Arugula [40g]
Asparagus [6 stems] {120g}
Avocado [2 3/4 hass]
Baby Spinach [2 cups] {80g}
Basil Leaves [25 leaves]
Broccoli [3 heads]
Brown Mushrooms [7]{70g}
Cauliflower [1 small]{300g}
Cherry Tomatoes [14]
Cilantro [1 stem]
Cucumber [3/4 cup] {85g}
Garlic [9 cloves]
Green Beans[50g]
Lettuce [18 leaves]
Parsley [2 stems]
Red Onion [1/16]
Red Pepper [3/4]
Swiss Chard [50g]
Tomato [4]
Zucchini [1 1/4]
Miscellaneous
Shirataki Noodles [200g]

WEEK 1

Day 1 - Make Ahead

1. **Savoury Breakfast Sausage**

185 calories 12.81g fat0.25g carbs0.2g fiber0.04g sugar16.17g protein

Mix all of the ingredients in a bowl and knead with
your hands.

Make six hamburger patty, wrap them in saran wrap and freeze them. We'll be using these for the next 6 days so if you think the meat will stay fresh, you don't have to freeze them, but I did just in case. I just thaw each hamburger the night before or thaw them in the microwave the day of.

Ingredients (6 portions) 220g ground chicken 220g ground pork

1tsp sage

1/2 tsp salt, thyme, black pepper 1/4 tsp celery seed, garlic powder, nutmeg, onion powder, paprika 1/8 tsp cayenne pepper

Day 1 - Breakfast
2. **Avocado Bun Breakfast Burger**

717 calories61.36g fat20.11g carbs 14.6g fiber2.88g sugar27.41g protein

Lay the avocado on its side, horizontally, and cut it right in the middle making sure you're not cutting it in an awkward angle. Once it's cut, carefully re- move the seed and carefully spoon out of the flesh. Cut the bottom of one avocado so that it can stand on its own on the plate.

Heat the oil in a non-stick skillet on medium-low heat. Add the breakfast sausage and cook 1-2 min- utes on each side until perfectly cooked. Crack the egg open in the skillet, turn the heat to low, cover and cook sunny side up. Cook for a couple of min- utes until the egg white is fully cooked.

Place the bottom half of the avocado on a plate, spoon some mayo in the avocado hole, top with lettuce, the tomato, sausage, carefully add the egg over and top wth the avocado top! Sprinkle some salt, pepper and sesame seeds.

Ingredients (1 portion)

1 avocado

1 egg

1tbsp olive oil 1breakfast sausage 1lettuce leaf

1slice tomato

1tbsp mayo

pinch salt, pepper, sesame seeds

3. **Avocado Cream & Zoodles**

383 calories 35.34g fat18g carbs9.4g fiber4.74g sugar5.46g protein

Spiralize your zucchini. Slice the mushrooms in
half.

In a stick blender cup, add the avocado, basil, 1tbsp olive oil, garlic, lemon juice and salt. Press the but- ton on the stick blender for about a minute until everything is super creamy and delicious.

Add 1/2 tbsp of olive oil in a frying pan and cook the mushrooms until tender. Add the zucchini noodles and cook just for a minute or so until they get hot.

Add the avocado cream, mix everything together

and serve.

Ingredients (1 portion)

1 zucchini

1/2 avocado (100g) 20 basil leaves

1.5 tbsp olive oil

3 brown mushrooms (30g) 1garlic clove

1tsp lemon juice 1/4 tsp salt

4. Chicken Cutlet & CauliRice

665 calories 42.35g fat14.64g carbs 8g fiber54. g sugar58.04g protein

Ingredients (2 portions)

Rice the cauliflower in a food processor or by using a cheese grater. In a wok, heat the sesame oil and add the riced cauliflower. Fry a couple of minutes, add the coconut aminos, dashi, salt and pepper, and mix until combined. Fry until the cauliflower is soft and crunchy.

Crush the pork rinds using a food processor/coffee grinder/or your hands. Mix the rinds with the al- mond flour, salt and pepper. Add the egg in a small bowl and whisk.

Slice the chicken breast in 2 lenght ways. Sprinkle the salt and pepper on both sides and dip in it the whisked egg. Coat the chicken with the breading on both sides.

Fry the cutlet in 150C/300F preheated oil and fry until the inner temperature of the chciken cutlet registers to 65C/150F. Serve with the cauli rice. Keep half for another meal.

small cauliflower (300g)

tbsp sesame oil 1tbsp coconut aminos 1tsp dashi powder

1/4 tsp salt + pepper

1skinless chicken breast (260g)

pinch salt + pepper

1 egg

4 tbsp almond flour 40g pork rinds pinch salt + pepper
frying oil (refined coconut oil/lard/ beef tallow)

5. **Breakfast Sausage, Eggs & Greens**

560 calories 43.30g fat12g carbs7g fiber2.79g sugar31.71g protein

Cut the stems off the green beans. Mince the garlic.

Put some water to boil in a pot. Add the broccoli and green beans and cook until tender. Take out of the water once cooked. Place the broccoli onto a plate.

Add the olive oil to a frying pan and add the break- fast sausage. Cook on both sides until cooked through. Add the eggs and scramble them. Place the eggs and sausage to the plate.

Add the garlic and green beans to the frying pan.

Fry until the garlic is starting to crisp up. Sprinkle

some salt, pepper and garlic powder over the beans and scrambled eggs. Place the beans and eggs onto the plate.

Ingredients (1 portion)

breakfast sausage

eggs

4 broccoli florets 50g green beans

1.5 tbsp olive oil 1garlic clove

pinch salt, pepper, garlic powder

6. **Chicken Cutlet & CauliRice**

665 calories 42.35g fat14.64g carbs 8g fiber4.54g sugar58.04g protein

Ingredients (2 portions)

1. Heat up the leftovers from last night's dinner!

2nd portion of Day 1 dinner!

7. Shirataki Noodles Asian Salad

149 calories 7.53g fat12.45g carbs 4.3g fiber5.02g sugar8.86g protein

Put some water to boil in a pot. Place the egg in- side and boil for 7 minutes exactly. Once cooked, transfer to a bowl full of ice water. Peel and cut in four.

Wash the shirataki noodles under some water and boil for 2 minutes. This will get rid of their smell. In the same pot, add the asparagus and boil until tender. Drain the water and let the noodles and

asparagus cool down. You can cut the noodles in half to make them shorter as they tend to be super long.

Thinly slice the red onion with a cabbage shredder. Cut the asparagus in half. Dice the tomato, slice the cucumber, chop the cilantro, and mince the

garlic using a garlic crusher.

Combine all of the ingredients in a large bowl and

mix. Serve cold!

Ingredients (1 portion)

200 g shirataki noodles (konjac) 2 asparagus (40g)

1/2 cup cucumber (65g)

1/2 tomato (65g) 1/16 red onions (20g) 1stem cilantro

1 garlic

egg

2tsp coconut aminos

1tsp fish sauce 1/2 tsp sesame oil 1tsp lemon juice

1/4 tsp salt and pepper

8. Breakfast Sausage & Eggs

477 calories 36.51g fat6.40g carbs2.5g fiber3.16g sugar30.61g protein

Cut the asparagus in two and cut off a bit off the

stems.

Put some water to boil and add the broccoli. Cook until tender.

Add 1/2 tbsp of olive oil to a non-stick frying pan and add the breakfast sausage and asparagus and cook on all sides until cooked through. Transfer to a plate with the boiled broccoli.

Add the other 1/2 tbsp of olive oil and crack the

eggs open. Switch the heat to low, cover and cook for a few minutes until the egg whites are fully cooked. Slide to the plate and sprinkle the salt, pepper and parsley over.

Ingredients (1 portion)

eggs

1breakfast sausage 1tbsp olive oil

asparagus

broccoli

3 cherry tomatoes

pinch salt, pepper, parsley

9. **BLT Lettuce Boats**

362 calories 33.20g fat10.64g carbs 3.34g fiber1.79g sugar8.62g protein

Fry the bacon in a frying pan until crispy.

Slice the tomato into a few slices. Slice the avo-

cado.

Spoon 1/2 tbsp of mayo over each lettuce leaf and cover with the bacon, tomato and avocado.

Ingredients (1 portion)

2 lettuce leaves

2 slices bacon 1/2 avocado 1/4 tomato

1tbsp mayo

10. **Grilled Cod & Shrimps**

338 calories 9.23g fat5.54g carbs1g fiber1.97g sugar55.42g protein

Mince the garlic and parsley

Melt the butter in a pan and add the garlic. Cook for a few seconds and place the cod and shrimp in the pan. Add the chopped parsley. Cook the shrimps for a few minutes until they turn orange. For the cod, cook for 2 minutes on each side, carefully not breaking it apart when flipping it over. Add the

tomatoes to the pan and fry with the shrimps for about a minute until soft.

Add the lemon juice over everything and it's ready

to serve. Store half for tomorrow.

Ingredients (2 portions) 2 cod fillet (300g)

200g shrimps

tbsp lemon juice 2stems fresh parsley 2 tbsp olive oil

garlic cloves

8 cherry toamtoes

11. **Easy Dairy-free CaesarDressing**

106 calories 11.39g fat0.4g carbs0.1g fiber0.02g sugar0.32g protein

1. Mince the garlic. Mix all of the ingredients together

and keep in an air-tight container in the fridge. It will keep for weeks, just mix it again before using.

Ingredients (6 portions)

6 tbsp mayonnaise 2tsp anchovy paste 1garlic clove

3tbsp unsweetened almond milk 1/2 tsp lemon juice

1.5 tsp oregano 1/8 tsp salt

1/4 tsp garlic powder

12. 9 0 sec Sausage Egg McMuffin

719 calories60.15g fat9.38g carbs4.15g fiber2.61g sugar36.57g protein

Combine the ingredients for the 90 second bread into a large mug. Mix carefully and microwave for 90 seconds. Take it out of the mug and carefully

slice in half.

Heat the olive oil in a frying pan and fry the break- fast sausage until cooked. Add the sliced bread and grill on both sides until desired toastness.

Using a mini egg frying pan, cook the egg until the

egg whites are fully cooked.

Spread the mayo over one slice of bread, cover with the tomato slice, sausage, egg and last slice of bread. Enjoy!!

Ingredients (1 portion) 1breakfast sausage 1slice tomato

1 egg

1tsp olive oil 1tsp mayo

90 sec bread: mix all of these

*1 tbsp refined coconut oil

*1 egg

*1/2 tsp salt

*1/2 tsp baking powder

*3 tbsp almond flour

13. Grilled Cod & Shrimps

338 calories 9.23g fat5.54g carbs1g fiber1.97g sugar55.42g protein

1. Reheat yesterday's dinners leftover and enjoy!

Ingredients (2 portions) Leftovers from Day 3 Dinner

14. **Arugula Caesar Salad & Veggies**

259 calories 19.62g fat19.08g carbs 9.1g fiber7.34g sugar7.07g protein

Put some water to boil and cook the broccoli and

asparagus until tender.

Shred the ruccola and iceberg lettuce and put into a bowl.

Slice the avocado, tomato, and cucumber. Put ev-

erything in a plate and cover with the dressing.

Ingredients (1 portion)

3 leaves iceberg lettuce (120g) 40g arugula

2 asparagus (60g)

4 broccoli florets (60g)

5-6 slices cucumber (20g)

1/2 avocado

1/2 tomato

1portion caesar dressing

15. **Breakfast Sausage & Poached Egg**

461 calories 37.54g fat7.08g carbs4.2g fiber1.93g sugar24.55g protein

Put some water to heat in a small pot and add the vinegar. Crack the egg inside a small bowl or cup. Once the water is simmering, make a circulating motion with a spatula inside the water and drop the egg in the middle of the spiral. Turn off the heat, cover for 6 minutes exactly. Take it out of the water once done.

Heat the olive oil in a frying pan and cook the breakfast sausage on medium-low heat on both sides until cooked through. Place the sausage on a plate. Add the fresh spinach to the frying pan with the leftover grease from the sausage. Cook

until wilted and transfer to a plate. Cover with the poached egg.

Slice the avocado and put on the plate along with the cherry tomatoes.

Ingredients (1 portion) 1breakfast sausage 1tbsp olive oil

egg

40g fresh spinach 3 cherry tomatoes 1/4 avocado

1/4 tsp salt & pepper 1tbsp vinegar

16. Rosemary Chicken & Broccoli

461 calories 33.71g fat6.99g carbs2.8g fiber1.7g sugar33.94g protein

Cut the chicken leg into bite-size pieces. Sprinkle the salt and pepper all over it. Separate the broccoli into florets.

In a cast iron skillet, heat the olive oil and add the chicken skin side down to the pan along with the rosemary. Fry 3 minutes to crisp up the skin and turn the chicken around. Add the broccoli florets and cook for a minute mixing everything together. Add the water, cover and let the steam of the water cook the broccoli for 2 minutes. Uncover and serve.

Ingredients (1 portion) 1boneless chicken leg (125g) 1/3 broccoli head (100g)

1/4 tsp salt

1/4 tsp black pepper 1/2 tsp rosemary 1tbsp olive oil

tbsp water

17. Rosemary Pork Roast

359 calories 23.88g fat0.12g carbs0.1g fiber0g sugar 33.75g protein

Preheat the oven to 200C/400F.

Massage the olive oil, salt, black pepper and rose- mary into the pork roast. Place it on a baking tray over some parchment paper.

Place in the oven and cook 1hour. Take it out and let cool for 5-10 minutes. Slice and serve. Keep 2/3 for the other meals.

Ingredients (3 portions) 500g boneless pork roast 1tbsp olive oil

1tsp salt

1tsp black pepper

1tbsp rosemary

18. Side Caesar Salad 3

214 calories 16.72g fat7.85g carbs2.6g fiber3.66g sugar8.96g protein

Put some water to boil and add the egg. Boil for 7 minutes exactly, transfer to an bowl filled with ice water. Peel it. Put the broccoli to boil and cook until tender.

Slice the broccoli and egg. Rip the lettuce leaves.

Mix everything together with the caesar dress- ing and eat with one portion of the rosemary pork roast.

Ingredients (1 portion)

4 lettuce leaves

1 egg

1/2 tomato

3 broccoli stems (50g)

1 tbsp caesar dressing

19. **Spinach & Pork Omelette**

446 calories 34.96g fat4.29g carbs0.9g fiber3.39g sugar27.84g protein

Crumble the sausage. Slice the red pepper and

mince the garlic.

In a large non-stick frying pan, add the olive oil and cook the sausage. Add the garlic, red pepper and

spinach to the pan and cook for 1-2 minutes until

soft.

Crack the eggs open in a large bowl, add the spices and mix with a whisk for 2 minutes.

Pour the egg batter to the pan, cover and let cook on low heat for 4-5 minutes.

When the top of the omeltte is cooked through, just slide the omelette to a plate and cut in half. Save half for the next day.

Ingredients (2 portions) 1breakfast sausage 1cup fresh spinach (30g)

1/4 red pepper (40g) 2garlic cloves

2 tbsp olive oil

1/4 tsp salt, pepper, garlic powder, parsley

6 eggs

20. **Rosemary Pork Roast**

359 calories 23.88g fat0.12g carbs0.1g fiber0g sugar33.75g protein

1. Reheat 1/3 of the pork roast from Day 5 dinner.

Ingredients (3 portions) Leftovers from Dinner 5 Dinner

21. **Side Caesar Salad2**

264 calories 19.15 fat6.64g carbs2g fiber4.19g sugar16.32g protein

Put some water to boil and add the egg. Boil for 7 minutes exactly, transfer to an bowl filled with ice water. Peel it.

Slice the egg in four. Rip the lettuce leaves.

Mix everything together with the caesar dressing and eat with the leftover pork roast.

Ingredients (1 portion)

4 lettuce leaves 30g prosciutto 1 egg

1 tomato

1tbsp caesar dressing

22. **Bacon, Broccoli & Mushrooms**

386 calories 26.22g fat4g carbs1.6g fiber0.98g sugar32.72g protein

Put some water to boil in a small pot and cook the

broccoli until tender.

Sprinkle the salt over the bacon slices and cut into 1cm strips.

Cut the mushrooms in 6.

Fry the bacon in a frying pan for a minute and add the mushrooms. Add the rosemary and fry until the bacon is crispy. Add the broccoli, mix everything together and sprinkle the garlic podwer and black pepper over.

Ingredients (1 portion) 80g broccoli

brown mushrooms (40g) 3 slices bacon (40g cooked) 1/4 tsp salt

1/2 tsp rosemary

1/4 tsp garlic powder pinch black pepper.

23. Spinach & Pork Omelette

446 calories 34.96g fat4.29g carbs0.9g fiber3.39g sugar27.84g protein

1. Reheat Day 6's breakfast leftovers.Ingredients (2 portions)

leftovers from Day 6 breakfast

24. Zucchini Salad w/ Grilled Chicken Thigh

430 calories 36.93g fat8.18g carbs2.6g fiber3.89g sugar17.84g protein

Using a peeler, peel the zucchini lenghtwise to

make long ribbons. Slice the red pepper and cut in half. Dice the tomato. Chop the swiss chard. Mince the basil leaves and garlic cloves.

Mix all of the above with the olive oil, vinegar and

salt & pepper together in a bowl and put on a plate.

Sprinkle the salt and pepper over the chicken thigh. Preheat the oil in a cast iron skillet and place chicken breast skin-side down and cook until crispy. Turn it around, cook a few more minutes until cooked through. Place on the plate with the salad.

Ingredients (1 portion)

1/4 zucchini

1/4 red pepper 50g swiss chard 1/4 tomato

basil leaves 1tbsp olive oil 1tsp vinegar

1 garlic clove

1/4 tsp salt & pepper

1chicken thigh with skin (75g) 1tbsp olive oil

1/2 tsp salt & pepper

25. Rosemary Pork Roast

359 calories 23.88g fat0.12g carbs0.1g fiber0g sugar33.75g protein

1. Reheat the leftovers from Day 5's dinner and serve

with the side caesar salad 1.

Ingredients (3 portions) leftovers from Day 5 Dinner

26. Side Caesar Salad1

274 calories 19.21g fat8.83g carbs2.2g fiber3g sugar16.94g protein

Put some water to boil and add the egg. Boil for 7 minutes exactly, transfer to an bowl filled with ice water. Peel it. Put the broccoli to boil and cook until tender.

Slice the broccoli and egg. Rip the lettuce leaves.

Slice the tomato and red pepper.

Mix everything together with the caesar dress- ing and eat with one portion of the rosemary pork roast.

Ingredients (1 portion)

4 lettuce leaves 30g prosciutto 1 egg

1/2 tomato

1/4 red pepper

2 broccoli stems (25g)

1tbsp caesar dressing

Week 2 Menu

	Breakfast	Lunch	Dinner	Nutritional Info
Day 8	Avocado Boat, Sausage & Asparagus	Rosemary Shrimps & Radishes	Chicken Brochettes and Sesame Salad	1266 calories 91.45g fat 16.02g net carbs 8.52g sugars 81.77g protein
Day 9	Eggs, Bacon & Tomato Salad	Chicken Brochettes & Easy Sesame Salad	Lettuce-wrapped Burger	1299 calories 97.34g fat 16.86g net carbs 11.5g sugars 80.22g protein
Day 10	Avocado Boat, Sausages, & Scrambled Eggs	Chicken Brochettes & Sesame Salad	Arugula Salad with Basil Vinaigrette	1529 calories 120.89g fat 19.48g net carbs 10.59g sugars 40.37g protein
Day 11	Fluffy Omelette & Veggies	Zucchini & Cucumber Salad	Roasted Chicken Leg & Veggies	1191 calories 83g fat 19.08g net carbs 13.48g sugars 85.18g protein
Day 12	Grilled Veggies & Fluffy Omelette	Roasted Chicken Leg & Veggies Leftovers	Cauliflower & Veggie Ranch Salad	1434 calories 103.26g fat 19.79g net carbs 14.77g sugars 97.3g protein
Day 13	Veggie Omelette	Kale Beef & Veggie Caesar Wrap	Grilled Rosemary Chicken with Veggies	1779calories 125.69g fat 20.33g net carbs 9.46g sugars 92.39g protein

Day 14 34	Eggs in Mini Skillet	Grilled Rosemary Chicken with Veggies Leftovers	Grilled Chicken & Guacamole	1834 calories 130.48g fat 17.71gnet carbs 9.11g sugars 95.34g protein

Week 2 Grocery List

Canned Goods
Tuna [140g]
Condiments
Coconut Aminos [37 ml]
Lemon Juice [15 ml]
Mayonnaise [112 ml]
Tahini [15 ml] (sesamepaste)
White Vinegar [20 ml]
Dairy
Almond Milk Unsweetened [5 ml]
Eggs [14]
Fruits
Lemon [2]
Meat
Bacon [7 slices]
Breakfast Pork Sausage [5] {200g}
Chicken Leg [4] {1100g} boneless
Chicken Leg [2] {600g} bone-in
Chicken Thigh [1] {150g} withskin
Ground Beef [70g]
Prosciutto [60g]
Thinly Sliced Beef[100g]
Oil
Chili Oil [1/4tsp]
Olive Oil [205 ml]
Sesame Oil [15 ml]
Spices
Black Pepper
Chili Powder
Cumin Powder
Garlic Powder

Himalayan Salt
Onion Powder
Oregano
Paprika Powder
Parsley
Rosemary
Sesame Seeds
Stevia Powder [1/16 tsp]
Thyme
Vegetables
Arugula [40g]
Asparagus [12 stems] {320g}
Avocado [3 hass]
Basil Leaves [11]
Black Olives [2 tbsp]
Brown Mushrooms [10]
Broccoli [2 heads]
Cauliflower [3 florets]
Cherry Tomatoes [18 cherries]
Cucumber [1 cup]
Garlic [16]
Kale [1 leaf] {50g}
Lettuce [16 leaves]
Long Asian Green Onion [1] (JapaneseLeek)
Mini Carrots [1 bag] (about200g)
Okra [2]
Radishes [15]
Red Onion [1/2]
Red Pepper [1 1/2]
Spinach [4 1/4 cups]
Spring Onions [2 stems]
Swiss Chard [30g]
Tomato [4]
Zucchini [1 1/2]

Day 8 - Breakfast

1. **Avocado Boat, Sausage & Asparagus**

537 calories 42.29g fat11.2g carbs8.3g fiber1.3g sugar30.78g protein
Heat the olive oil in a small frying pan and fry the sausages and asparagus until cooked through. Transfer to a plate.
Scoop the inside of the avocado and place it in a bowl, along with the tuna, wilted spinach, mayo and salt & pepper. Stuff the avocado shell with it and place on the plate.
Ingredients (1 portion) 60g sausage
1-2 asparagus 1tsp olive oil 1/2 avocado 70g tuna
1/4 cup wilted spinach (50g fresh) 1tbsp mayo
pinch salt & pepper

Day 8 - Lunch
2. **Rosemary Shrimps & Radishes**

261 calories15.63g fat8.13g carbs3.2g fiber2.82g sugar22.64g protein

Put some water to boil in a pot and add the broccoli. Cook until tender.

In a skillet, heat the oil and add the radishes to one side and the shrimps to another. Sprinkle the salt, pepper and rosemary and cook for a few minutes.

The radishes should be soft and crunchy, and the
shrimps should be orange.

Put everything on a plate and enjoy!

Ingredients (1 portion)

5 radishes (85g)

10 shrimps (100g)

3 broccoli florets (60g) 1tbsp rosemary

1tbsp olive oil

1/2 tsp salt, pepper

3. **Soy & Dairy-free Creamy Sesame Dressing**

61 calories5.95g fat1.27g carbs1g fiber0g sugar0.42g protein

1. Mix all of the ingredients together in a small bowl. Store in an air-tight container in the fridge. Just remix with a spoon before use each time.

Ingredients (10 portions)

3 tbsp mayo

2.5 tbsp coconut aminos 1tbsp sesame oil

1tbsp tahini

1tbsp crushed sesame seeds 1tbsp sesame seeds

1tsp vinegar

1/16 tsp stevia powder

4. Chicken & VegetableBrochettes

317 calories20.11g fat7.21g carbs1.5g fiber2.79g sugar26.35g protein

Preheat the oven to 210C/420F.

Dice the chicken leg into bite size pieces. Slice the long green onion into 12-14 pieces. Cut the aspara- gus into 4.

Add all of the ingredients to a bowl and mix togeth- er. Skewer the veggies and chicken on 9 brochettes.

Place in the oven and bake for 20 minutes.

Ingredients (3 portions) 1boneless chicken leg (300g) 4 asparagus

1large asian green onion

1tbsp lemon juice from a lemon 1tbsp rosemary

10 cherry tomatoes 1tbsp olive oil 1tsp salt & pepper 5 garlic cloves

1/2 tsp onion powder

5. Chicken Brochettes & SesameSalad

468 calories 33.53g fat14.89g carbs 6.7g fiber4.44g sugar28.35g protein

Rip the lettuce into bite size pieces. Scoop out the avocado and cube it, slice the tomato slice in a few pieces. Add the sesame dressing and coat well.

Add the brochettes to a plate along with the salad.

Ingredients (1 portion)
3 chicken & veggie brochettes 3 lettuce leaves
1tomato slice
1/4 avocado
1portion sesame dressing

6. Eggs, Bacon & Tomato Salad

541 calories 39.81g fat8.12g carbs1.8g fiber4.42g sugar36.3g protein
Slice the red pepper and zucchini.
Fry the bacon in a small non-stick frying pan until crispy. Put the bacon on a plate. Fry the peppers and zucchini in the bacon fat until tender, crack the eggs open and scramble until cooked. Sprinkle the salt and pepper over. Put on the plate with the bacon.
Mince the garlic clove and basil leaf. Mix the olive oil, basil, garlic, vinegar, salt & pepper together in a small bowl. Add the tomato slices to the plate and pour the dressing over.
Ingredients (1 portion)
3 slices bacon
eggs
1/4 red pepper 1/4 zucchini (40g)
pinch salt & pepper
slices tomato
1basil leaf 1tsp olive oil 1garlic clove
1/2 tsp vinegar
sprinkle salt & pepper

7. Chicken Brochettes & Easy Salad

400 calories 26.29g fat13.28g carbs 4.2g fiber5.89g sugar27.92g protein

Rip the lettuce into bite size pieces. Slice the red pepper and tomato. Add the sesame dressing and coat well.

Add the brochettes to a plate along with the salad.

Ingredients (1 portion)

3 chicken brochettes

5 lettuce leaves 1/4 red pepper 1slice tomato

1tbsp sesame dressing

8. **Lettuce-wrapped Burger**

358 calories 31.24g fat2.76g carbs1.3g fiber1.19g sugar16g protein

Fry the bacon in a skillet until crispy. Form a ham- burger patty with the ground beef and fry in the leftover bacon grease. Cook on both sides until cooked through.

Add the spinach to the leftover grease in the skillet and cook until wilted.

Add the mayo, tomato, spinach, patty and bacon in

a large lettuce leaf, fold and make a burger!

Ingredients (1 portion)

70g ground beef

slices bacon (50g) (18g cooked) 1large lettuce leaf

1cup fresh baby spinach

9. 1slice tomato 1tbsp mayo

10. **Basil Vinaigrette**

188 calories 20.28g fat2.27g carbs0.2g fiber0.24g sugar0.38g protein

1. Crush the garlic cloves using a garlic crusher. Mince the basil leaves. Combine all of the ingre- dients into a bowl and mix. Refrigerate until later used.

Ingredients (2 portions) 3 tbsp olive oil

1tbsp white vinegar 1tbsp lemon juice

garlic cloves

10 basil leaves

1/4 tsp salt, pepper

11. Avocado Boat, Sausages & Scrambled Eggs

792 calories 64.82g fat11.23g carbs 7.5g fiber2.19g sugar42.93g protein

Slice the mushrooms.

Heat the oil in a small non stick frying pan and fry the sausages. Once cooked, add them to a plate. Fry the mushrooms and fresh spinach until soft and add the eggs. Scramble until cooked, sprinkle the

salt and pepper, and add to the plate.

Scoop out the insides of the avocado, and mix with the green onions, tuna, mayo and salt and pepper in a small bowl. Refill the avocado shell with the bowl ingredients and place on the plate.

Ingredients (1 portion)

60g sausage

2 eggs

mushrooms 1/4 spinach 1tbsp olive oil

pinch salt & pepper 1/2 avocado

70g tuna can

1tbsp mayo

1tsp sliced green onion pinch salt & pepper

12. Chicken Brochettes & SesameSalad

468 calories 33.53g fat14.89g carbs 6.7g fiber4.44g sugar28.35g protein

Rip the lettuce into bite size pieces. Scoop out the avocado and cube it, slice the tomato slice in a few pieces. Add the sesame dressing and coat well.

Add the brochettes to a plate along with the salad.

Ingredients (1 portion)

chicken & veggie brochettes 3 lettuce leaves

1tomato slice

1/4 avocado

1tbsp sesame dressing

13. Arugula salad with Basil Vinaigrette

269 calories 22.54g fat10.46g carbs 2.9g fiber3.96g sugar9.09g protein

Put some water to boil in a pot and add the broc- coli. Cook until tender and cool under cold water.

In a bowl, mix all of the ingredients together and

serve on a plate!

Ingredients (1 portion)

40g arugula

1/2 tomato

5-6 slices cucumber

slices prosciutto (20g)

broccoli florets (50g)

1serving Basil Vinaigrette

14. **Fluffy Omelette & Veggies**

263 calories 19.29g fat8.56g carbs2.4g fiber5.26g sugar14.98g protein

Crack the eggs open in a bowl and beat with a hand mixer for 3 minutes.

Add 1tsp of olive oil to a non-stick pan and pour the whipped eggs in. Cover and cook on low heat for about 2 minutes, or until the eggs are cooked through. This will be a fluffy omelette. Fold in half and slide onto a plate.

Dice the red pepper, slice the mushrooms and chop the swiss chard. Heat the oil in a non-stick frying pan and add the red peppers. Cook for a minute, add the mushrooms and swiss chard and cook until wilted. Sprinkle the salt, pepper and garlic powder. Place over the folded omelette.

Ingredients (1 portion)

1/2 red pepper 30g swiss chard 3 mushrooms

tsp olive oil

pinch salt, pepper, garlic powder

eggs

1tsp olive oil

15. **Fluffy Omelette & Veggies**

296 calories 25.93g fat9.16g carbs2.3g fiber3.53g sugar9.05g protein

Using a cabbage shredder, thinly slice the zucchini and cucumber.

Chop the spinach and cut the egg in 4.

Place everything on a plate and pour the dressing over.

Ingredients (1 portion)

1/2 zucchini (100g) 1/2 small cucumber 1/2 cup fresh spinach 1hard-boiled egg

1serving basil vinaigrette

16. Roasted Chicken Leg & Veggies

632 calories 37.78g fat9.06g carbs3g fiber4.69g sugar61.15g protein

Ingredients (2 portions)

Preheat the oven to 200C/400F.

Cut the stems off the asparagus. Slice the zucchini into vertical slices. Slice the mini carrots in half.

Place all of the veggies in a 10" cast iron skillet. Cover with the two chicken legs. Pour the olive oil over everything. Sprinkle the spices over both of the chicken legs.

Place the skillet in the oven and bake for 50 min- utes uncovered.

Take out and enjoy. Keep half for another meal.

6 asparagus spears (40g)

1/2 zucchini

100g mini carrots

2 chicken legs (600g) 1tbsp olive oil

6 cherry tomatoes (80g)

1/4 tsp salt, black pepper, cumin, paprika, chili powder

17. Grilled Veggies & FluffyOmelette

492 calories 42.26g fat8.37g carbs2.2g fiber5.38g sugar21.16g protein

Crack the eggs open in a bowl and beat with a hand

mixer for 3 minutes.

Dice the red pepper, slice the mushrooms and slice the mushrooms. Heat 1tbsp of olive oil in a non-

stick frying pan and add the red peppers. Cook for a minute, add the mushrooms and spinach and cook until wilted. Sprinkle the salt, pepper and

garlic powder. Set aside.

Add 1tbsp of olive oil to a non-stick pan and pour the whipped eggs in. Cover and cook on low heat for about 2 minutes, or until the eggs are cooked through. This will be a fluffy omelette. Place the cooked veggies on one side of the omelette and fold in half. Carefully slide onto a plate.

Ingredients (1 portion) 1/2 red pepper

1/2 cup fresh spinach 3 mushrooms

2 tbsp olive oil

pinch salt, pepper, garlic powder 3 eggs

18. Roasted Chicken Leg & Veggies

632 calories 37.78g fat9.06g carbs3g fiber4.69g sugar61.15g protein

Ingredients (2 portions)

1. Leftovers from Day 11's dinner.

Leftovers from Day 11's Dinner.

19. Cauliflower & Veggie Ranch Salad

310 calories 23.22g fat12.32g carbs 4.76g fiber4.7g sugar14.90g protein
Ingredients (1 portion)
Put some water to boil in a pot and add the cauliflower and broccoli in. Cook until tender.
Cut the tomato and slice the cucumber.
Mix the dressing ingredients together.
Add all of the salad ingredients on a plate and
drizzle the dressing over.
4 lettuce leaves
3 broccoli florets (50g)
3 cauliflower florets (50g) 40g prosciutto
1/2 tomato
1/4 cup sliced cucumber
2 tbsp sliced black olives
Spicy Ranch Dressing:
1.5 tbsp mayo
1tsp unsweetened almond milk
1/4 tsp paprika powder
1/4 tsp chili oil
1/4 tsp salt, pepper

20. **Veggie Omelette**

399 calories 27.97g fat9.34g carbs3.2g fiber4.42g sugar26.59g protein
Slice the broccoli, sausages, mushrooms, zucchini and cherry tomatoes in a few pieces.

Heat the oil in a medium skillet, and fry the sau- sage, mushrooms and zucchini slices for 2-3 min- utes until cooked through. Put aside.

Put some water to boil and boil the sliced broccoli and okra for 2 mintues. Take out of the boiling wa- ter, and slice the okra in 6-8 pieces.

Crack the eggs into a bowl and whisk for a minute with a whisk. Pour the egg batter in a frying pan and cook on low heat. Top with all of the veggies and meat, cover and cook until the eggs are cooked through. The omelette should just slide out of the frying pan onto a plate.

Ingredients (1 portion)

eggs

broccoli (40g)

okra (10g)

mushrooms (20g) 3breakfast sausage (80g) 1/4 zucchini (50g)

4cherry tomatoes 1tsp olive oil

pinch salt & pepper

21. Kale Beef & Veggie Caesar Wrap

714 calories59.64g fat17.23g carbs 8.6g fiber2.66g sugar30.93g protein

Carefully trim the stem of the kale leaf so that you

can roll the leaf to make a sandwich.

Slice the avocado, red onion and tomato.

Heat the olive oil in a skillet and add the sliced beef. Sprinkle the salt, pepper and garlic pow- der and cook until cooked through, 1-2 minutes.

Spoon the caesar dressing over the entire leaf. On one end, add all of the toppings and care- fully roll the leaf into a wrap. You can use aluminum foil to keep it from rolling out.

Ingredients (1 portion) 1portion caesar dressing 1large kale leaf (50g)

1/2 avocado 1/2 tomato 1/8 red onion

100g thinly sliced beef 1tbsp olive oil

1/4 tsp salt, pepper, garlic powder

22. Grilled Rosemary Chicken withVeggies

666 calories 38.08g fat7.76g carbs2.2g fiber2.38g sugar34.86g protein

Preheat the oven to 190C/410F.

Slice the radishes in half, cut the lemon into 6 slic- es, slice the red onion and cut the chicken thighs into two.

Place the chicken thighs on a baking tray that's

been covered with parchment paper (to avoid a

mess) and scatter the veggies everywhere around the thighs. Place the lemon slices over the chicken, drizzle the whole tray with the olive oil and sprinkle the salt, pepper, rosemary and thyme over every- thing.

Place in oven and bake for 45 minutes. Take out of the oven and serve hot!

Ingredients (3 portions)

boneless chicken legs (800g) 14 mini carrots

6 garlic cloves

10 radishes 1/4 red onion 1 lemon

1tbsp rosemary 1tbsp thyme 1/2 tsp salt

1/2 tsp black pepper

2 tbsp olive oil

23. Eggs in MiniSkillet

491 calories 40.87g fat15.07g carbs 8.7g fiber3.90g sugar19.34g protein

Ingredients (2 portions)

Fry the bacon until crispy in a 6" mini skillet. Chop into bits. Dice the tomato and avocado. Slice the okra into a few pieces.

In the same mini skillet, rack the eggs open into the bacon grease, cover and cook on low heat until cooked through. Top with the bacon bits, tomato, avocado, okra and broccoli. Sprinkle the salt, pepper and parsley over.

2 slices bacon

eggs

1/2 avocado 1 okra

1/2 tomato

3boiled broccoli (50g)

sprinkle salt, pepper, parsley

24. Grilled Rosemary Chicken withVeggies

666 calories 38.08g fat7.76g carbs2.2g fiber2.38g sugar34.86g protein

1. Heat up 1/3 of the leftovers from Day 13's dinner.Ingredients (3 portions)

leftover's from Day 13's dinner

25. Grilled Chicken & Guacamole

677 calories 51.53g fat14.38g carbs 8.6g fiber2.83g sugar41.14g protein

Sprinkle the salt and pepper over the chicken thigh on both sides.

Heat the olive oil in a cast iron skillet and place the thigh skin side down. Grill on both sides until cooked through, about 4-5 minutes.

Dice the tomato and red onion. Mince the garlic and green onion. Mash the avocado and mix with the rest, and add the salt and pepper. Top over chicken along with the broccoli.

Ingredients (1 portion) 1chicken thigh with skin(150g) 1tbsp olive oil

1/2 tsp salt, pepper

1/2 avocado

1/4 tomato

1green onion stem 1slice red onion pinch salt and pepper

boiled broccoli (25g)

Week 3

1. Week 3 Menu

	Breakfast	Lunch	Dinner	Nutritional Info
Day 15	Broccoli, Bacon & Poached Egg	Grilled Rosemary Chicken with Veggies Leftovers	Spicy Chicken & Kale Salad	1450 calories 91.88g fat 19.28g net carbs 8.4g sugars 89.73g protein
Day 16	Breakfast Egg Burrito	Spicy Chicken & Kale Salad Leftovers	Chicken Meatballs & Zoodles	1386 calories 98.37g fat 15.81g net carbs 13.24g sugars 88.56 protein
Day 17	Asparagus, Bacon & Poached Egg	Spicy Chicken & Kale Salad Leftovers	Cauli Mash & Chicken Meatballs	1165 calories 75.97g fat 21.19g net carbs 11.61g sugars 86.75g protein
Day 18	Bacon, Spinach & Eggs	Chicken Meatball Lettuce Cups	Chili Con Carne & Veggies	1318 calories 97.49g fat 19.2g net carbs 11.39g sugars 79.86g protein

Day 19	Bacon, Eggs & Asparagus	Chicken Meatball Lettuce Cups	Cauli Mash, Green Beans & Parsley Salmon	1376 calories 95.34g fat 19.19g net carbs 19.66g sugars 96.29g protein
Day 20	Chicken Meatballs & Eggs	Chili Con Carne	Grilled Salmon, Radishes & Green Beans	1277calories 85.05g fat 21.92g net carbs 12.96g sugars 97.14g protein
Day 21 60	Bacon, Spinach, Egg & Avocado	Chicken Meatballs & Arugula Salad	Chili Con Carne & Veggies + Egg	1376 calories 108.15g fat 20.34g net carbs 12.32g sugars 70.24g protein

2. Week 3 Grocery List

Baking
Blanched Almond Flour [70g]

Canned Goods
Diced Tomato Can [500 ml]
Tomato Paste [7 ml]

Condiments
Dijon Mustard [15ml]
Lemon Juice [25 ml]
Mayonnaise [40 ml]
White Vinegar [32 ml]

Dairy
Almond Milk Unsweetened [30 ml]

Egg [12]

Meat
Bacon [18 slices]
Chicken Breast [1] {285g} withskin
Ground Beef [200g]
Ground Chicken [650g]

Oil
Chili Oil [1/4 tsp] or cayenne pepper
Olive Oil [120 ml]

Seafood & Fish
Salmon Fillet [2] {300g}
Spices
Black Pepper
Chili Powder
Cumin Powder
Dill
Garlic Powder
Himalayan Salt
Onion Powder
Oregano
Paprika Powder
Parlsey
Rosemary
Sage
Thyme

Vegetables
Arugula [40g]
Asparagus [10 stems]{200g}
Avocado [3 hass]
Basil Leaves [10 leaves]
Black Olives [1 tbsp]
Broccoli [2 heads]
Brown Mushrooms [5]
Carrot [1/4]
Cauliflower [1 head]{300g}
Celery [1/2 stick]

Cherry Tomatoes [8 cherries]
Garlic [7 cloves]
Green Beans [150g]
Kale [6 leaves]{120g}
Lettuce [9 leaves]
Okra [2]
Onion [3/4]
Parsley [4 stems]
Radishes [5]
Red Cabbage [1/8]
Shiitake Mushrooms [3]
Spinach [1 cup]
Tomato [2]
Zucchini [1 1/2]

3.   Week 3

Day 15 - Breakfast

1.   Broccoli, Bacon & Poached Egg

378 calories 26.48g fat   11.46g carbs 4.6g fiber   2.76g sugar   23.99g protein

Put the broccoli to boil in a pot of water and cook until tender. Take the broccoli out and place on a plate.

In a different pot, add some water and the white vinegar and put to simmer. Add the egg in a bowl. Swirl the water with a spatula and add the egg in the middle of the whirlpool. Cover and turn off the heat and cook the egg for 6 minutes exactly. Care- fully take it out and place over the broccoli.

Fry the bacon in a skillet until crispy. Chop it up into a few pieces and place over the broccoli. Driz- zle the sesame dressing over everything. Sprinkle the salt, pepper and parsley.

Ingredients (1 portion)

1 egg

140g broccoli (1/3 head)

3 slices bacon (36g cooked) 1portion sesame dressing 1tbsp white vinegar

pinch salt, pepper, parsley

2.   Grilled Rosemary Chicken withVeggies

666 calories 38.08g fat   7.76g carbs   2.2g fiber   2.38g sugar   34.86g protein

1. Reheat 1/3 of the leftovers from Day 14's dinner.   Ingredients (3 portions)

1/3 leftover from day 14's dinner.

3.   *Spicy Chicken & KaleSalad*

406 calories 27.32g fat   9.96g carbs   3.1g fiber   3.26g sugar   30.88g protein

Slice the chicken breast in half lenght ways. Sprinkle the salt, pepper, paprika, cumin, garlic and oregano over the chicken breasts. Heat the 1tsp of olive oil on a grill or use a

Ingredients (3 portions) 1chicken breast (285g)

1/4 tsp salt, black pepper,

Spicy Salad Dressing: 2 tbsp mayo

1tbsp lemon juice

bbq, and grill your chicken 4-5 minutes until

cooked through. Slice in 5-6 pieces.

paprika, cumin, garlic pow-   1tbsp olive oil

Slice lenghtways the zucchini. Heat the 1 tbsp of olive oil in a non-stick frying pan and add

der

1tsp oregano

1/2 tsp vinegar

1/2 tsp paprika powder

the zucchini slices. Sprinkle the salt and pep- 2 tsp olive oil

per over and grill on both sides until browned.

1/8 tsp salt

Boil the broccoli and okras for 2 minutes. Us-

small kale leaves (120g)

1/4 tsp garlic powder

ing a cabbage shredder, shred the red cab-

bage and thinly slice the watermelon radish.

6-7 broccoli with stem (100g)1 tsp oregano

Shred with your hands the kale.

In a small bowl, combine the salad dressing

ingredients.

On a large plate, cover with the kale, the rest of the veggies, and grilled chicken. Pour 1/3 of the spicy dressing over ONE portion.

Place the rest in some tupperwares for the

64 next 2 meals and keep the dressing separated

2 okra (20g)

100g red cabbage (1/8) 8 cherry tomatoes (65g) 4-5 radishes

1/2 zucchini (70g) 1tbsp olive oil

1/4 tsp hili oil or cay- enne pepper

4. Breakfast Egg Burrito

538 calories 46.85g fat 10.35g carbs 6.9g fiber   1.96g sugar   20.7g protein

In a Japanese rectangular tamagoyaki frying pan, heat 1/2 tsp of olive oil. In a small bowl, whisk the two eggs together for 20 seconds or so. Pour half of the eggs into the pan, spread out evenly and cook on medium-low heat until the egg is cooked through. Carefully slide onto a plate. Repeat this step with the leftover egg mixture.

Fry the bacon until crispy.

Slice the avocado in a few slices. Slice the tomato in two. Chop the lettuce.

On each egg omelette, spread 1/2 tbsp of mayo. Cover with the lettuce, tomato, avocado and bacon and carefully roll up like a burrito.

Ingredients (1 portion)

eggs

1tsp olive oil 2 slices bacon 1lettuce leaf 1/2 avocado

1slice tomato 1tbsp mayo

5. Spicy Chicken & KaleSalad

406 calories 27.32g fat   9.96g carbs   3.1g fiber   3.26g sugar   30.88g protein

Drizzle 1/2 of the dressing over 1/2 of the left- Ingredients (3 portions)

overs from day 15's dinner and enjoy!

Spicy Salad Dressing:

leftover from day 15's dinner leftover from day 15's

dinner.

6. Chicken & Herbs Meatballs

442 calories 28.34g fat   6.47g carbs   2.2g fiber   1.64g sugar   40.12g protein

Preheat the oven to 200C/400F.

Mince the garlic, shiitake and onion.

Add the olive oil to a frying pan and fry the mush- rooms, onions and garlic until tender. Turn off heat and transfer to a bowl.

Mix all of the remaining ingredients into a large bowl and mix until well incorporated.

Place a parchment paper over a baking tray. Make 12 large meatballs and place them on the baking tray carefully making space between each meatball. The mixture is a bit sticky, but that's fine. It'll cook perfectly in the oven.

Add to the oven and cook for 25 minutes. Take out and let cool before keeping them in the fridge.

Ingredients (6 portions)

shiitake mushrooms (60g) 1/2 white onion (90g)

2 garlic cloves 1tsp olive oil

650g ground chicken

2-3 stems chopped parsley (8g)

10 leaves chopped basil (5g)

1tsp thyme, sage

1/2 tsp onion powder, salt, pepper

1/4 tsp garlic powder

1 egg

70g blanched almond flour

7.   Chicken Meatballs & Zoodles

423 calories 24.2g fat 17.6g carbs   12.1g fiber

Spiralize your zucchini. Cut the meatballs into 8.

Add the tomatoes, water and spices to a pot and simmer for 5-10 minutes until desired thickness. Add the meat to the tomato sauce, mix well

Add the zoodles to the sauce and cook for a minute or so just to get them warmed up.

8.02g sugar   36.98g protein

Ingredients (1 portion)

2 chicken meatballs

zucchini

1/2 cup diced tomato can

1/2 cup water

1/4 tsp garlic powder, onion power, basil, parsley, oregano

8. Asparagus, Bacon & Poached Egg

288 calories 21.07g fat   6.65g carbs   3.15g fiber   2.64g sugar   18.21g protein

Add some water to a small pot and the white vine- gar and put to simmer. Add the egg in a bowl. Swirl the water with a spatula and add the egg inside the middle of the whirlpool. Turn off the heat and cook the egg for 6 minutes exactly. Carefully take it out.

Fry the bacon until crispy. Cut the stems off the asparagus and fry into the bacon grease.

Place the asparagus onto a plate, cover with the bacon and poached egg and spoon the sesame dressing over. Add a bit of parlsey over everything.

Ingredients (1 portion)

6 asparagus

3 slices bacon

1 egg

1tbsp sesame dressing 1tbsp white vinegar pinch parsley

9. Spicy Chicken & KaleSalad

406 calories 27.32g fat   9.96g carbs   3.1g fiber   3.26g sugar   30.88g protein

Drizzle 1/2 of the dressing over 1/2 of the left- Ingredients (3 portions)   Spicy Salad Dressing: overs from day 15's dinner and enjoy!

leftover from day 15's dinner leftover from day 15's dinner.

10. Cauli Mash & ChickenMeatballs

471 calories   27.81g fat   18.45g carbs 7.46g fiber

Mince the garlic cloves.

Separate the cauliflower florets. Put some water to boil in a large pot and cover with a metal steamer. Add the cauliflower, cover, and cook for 5-7 minutes until tender. Once tender, transfer to a small bowl, add half the garlic, almond milk, garlic powder, onion powder, 1/2 tsp of salt and pepper. Using a

stick blender (or a food processor), puree the cauliflower until desired consistency.

Put the green beans to a boil and cook for 5-6 min- utes. Take out of the water into a frying pan along with the olive oil and add the leftover minced gar- lic. Sprinkle the 1/4 tsp of salt and pepper over and cook in the frying pan until the garlic gets crispy.

Reheat two chicken meatballs and place on a plate with half the cauliflower mash and half the green beans. Add the parsley over the cauli mash. Keep the other half for tomorrow.

5.71g sugar   37.66g protein

Ingredients (1 portion)

chicken meatballs

Ingredients (2 portions) 1small cauliflower (300g) 3 garlic cloves

100g green beans

1/4 tsp salt

2tbsp unsweetened almond milk 2 tsp olive oil

1/4 tsp garlic powder, onion pow-

der

1/2 tsp salt, pepper pinch parsley

11. Bacon, Spinach & Eggs

354 calories 25.52g fat   2.39g carbs   0.7g fiber   0.9g sugar   27.14g protein

Fry the bacon until crispy.

Chop the spinach and add to the frying pan where the bacon was. Cook in the bacon grease until wilted. Crack the eggs open over the spinach, cover and cook for 2-3 minutes until the whites are fully cooked.

Sprinkle the salt and pepper over the eggs. Slide down onto a plate with the bacon.

Ingredients (1 portion)

slices bacon (40g cooked) 2 eggs

30g spinach

pinch salt, pepper

12. Chicken Meatball Lettuce Cups

599 calories 44.65g fat   17.04g carbs 9.6g fiber   3.73g sugar   36.57g protein

Dice the tomato and avocado. Cut the meatballs into four pieces. Place two lettuce leaves on top of each other.

Mix the mayo and dijon in a small bowl. Spread half on each cup.

Add half the meatballs, tomato and avocado to
each lettuce cup. Add a bit of chopped parsley over everything.
Ingredients (1 portion)
lettuce leaves
2 chicken meatballs 1/4 tomato
1/2 avocado 1/2 tbsp mayo 1/2 tbsp dijon
pinch of parsley

13. *Chili Con Carne*

281 calories 19.91g fat
g carbs 3.6g fiber   5.9g sugar   14.97g protein
Ingredients (3 portions)
Dice the onion, celery and carrot. Slice the mushrooms. Mince the garlic.
Add the olive oil to a large pot and add all of the
veggies. Cook for 3-4 minutes until tender. Add the ground beef and cook until browned. Add
the rest of the ingredients and mix to combine. Put on low
heat and simmer for 10-15 minutes until desired thickness.
74
1/4 small white onion (35)
1/2 celery stick (5g) 50g brown mushrooms 1/4 carrot (50g)
1garlic clove
tbsp olive oil
200g ground beef
1.5 cups diced tomato can (400g)
1/2 cup water
1tbsp chili powder
1/2 tbsp oregano, tomato paste 3/4 tsp cumin ground
1/2 tsp thyme
1/4 tsp salt, pepper
1/8 tsp cayenne pepper, garlic powder, onion powder

14. Chili Con Carne & Veggies

365 calories 27.32g fat   17.47g carbs 7.2gfiber 6.76g sugar   16.15g protein
Ingredients (1 portion)
Top 1/3 of the chili with sliced avocado and diced tomato. Enjoy!
1/3 portion chili 1/4 avocado 1slice tomato

15. Bacon, Eggs &Asparagus

370 calories 27.90g fat   8.3g carbs   5.1g fiber
Cut the stems off the asparagus. Slice the avocado. Put some water to boil in a pot and add the aspara- gus. Cook until tender.
Fry the bacon in a skillet until crispy.
Crack the egg in the bacon grease and cook it until ready.
Add everything to the plate and sprinkle some salt and pepper over everything.
2.21g sugar   22.75g protein
Ingredients (1 portion) 1/4 avocado
bacon slices
asparagus
1 egg
pinch salt and pepper

16. Chicken Meatball Lettuce Cups

599 calories 44.65g fat   17.04g carbs 9.6g fiber   3.73g sugar   36.57g protein
Dice the tomato and avocado. Cut the meatballs into four pieces. Place two lettuce leaves on top of each other.
Mix the mayo and dijon in a small bowl. Spread half
on each cup.
Add half the meatballs, tomato and avocado to
each lettuce cup. Add a bit of chopped parsley over everything.
Ingredients (1 portion)
4 lettuce leaves
2 chicken meatballs 1/4 tomato
1/2 avocado 1/2 tbsp mayo 1/2 tbsp dijon
pinch of parsley

17. Cauli Mash, Green Beans & Parsley Salmon

407 calories 22.79g fat   14.48g carbs 5.93g fiber   4.72g sugar   36.97g protein

Reheat the cauli mash and green beans.

Mince the parsley sprig.

Rub the salmon filet with the olive oil, salt, pepper,
and parlsey.

Carefully place in a non-stick frying pan and cook on both sides for 2-3 minutes until perfectly cooked through. Once cooked, add the lemon juice over the salmon and serve with the veggies.

Ingredients (1 portion)

cauli mash leftovers from day 17 dinner

green beans leftovers from day 17

dinner

150g salmon filet 1sprig parsley 1tsp lemon juice 1tsp olive oil pinch salt, pepper

18. Chicken Meatballs & Eggs

581 calories 38.34g fat   11.48g carbs 3.7g fiber   4.33g sugar   47.87g protein

Put some water to boil in a small pot and add the broccoli. Cook until tender and add to a plate with the cherry tomatoes. Reheat the chicken meatballs and add to the plate.

Heat the olive oil in a frying pan and scramble the eggs until perfectly cooked. Sprinkle some salt and pepper over.

Ingredients (1 portion)

2 chicken meatballs

eggs

broccoli (50g)

3 cherry tomatoes 1tsp olive oil pinch salt, pepper

19. Chili Con Carne

281 calories 19.91g fat 12.4g carbs   3.6g fiber   5.9g sugar   14.97g protein

1. Reheat 1/3 of the chili and enjoy!

Ingredients (1 portion)
1/3 portion chili

20. Grilled Salmon, Radishes & Green Beans

415 calories 26.8g fat 9.04g carbs   3.7g fiber   2.73g sugar   34.3g protein

Rub the salmon with the oil, dill, salt and pepper.

Carefully place in a non-stick frying pan and cook on both sides for 2-3 minutes until perfectly cooked through. Once cooked, add the lemon juice over the salmon.

Mince the garlic clove. Put the green beans to a boil and cook for 5-6 minutes. Take out of the water into a frying pan along with the olive oil and add the minced garlic. Sprinkle the salt and pepper over and cook in the frying pan until the garlic gets crispy.

Heat the olive oil in a frying pan, add the radishes and the rosemary. Cook for 4-5 minutes until crispy. Sprinkle the salt and pepper.

Serve everything together on a plate and enjoy.

Ingredients (1 portion)
150g salmon fillet
1tsp olive oil
1/4 tsp dill, salt, black pepper
1tsp lemon juice
5 radishes (85g) 1tsp olive oil 1tbsp rosemary
pinch salt, pepper, garlic powder
50g green beans 1garlic clove
2 tsp olive oil

21. Bacon, Spinach, Egg &Avocado

347 calories 31.54g fat   5.76g carbs   4.1g fiber   0.84g sugar   11.51g protein

Fry the bacon in a skillet until crispy.

Add the spinach in the same skillet and cook in the bacon grease until wilted, and then transfer to a plate. Crack the egg in the bacon grease and cook until the white is cooked.

Slice the avocado. Put everything on a plate and sprinkle some salt and pepper over everything.

Ingredients (1 portion)
3 slices bacon

1 egg
30g spinach 1/4 avocado
pinch salt, pepper

22. Chicken Meatballs & ArugulaSalad

587 calories 44.01g fat   14.45g carbs 6.6g fiber

1. Slice the avocado, tomato and chicken meatballs. Put everything on a plate and drizzle the caesar dressing over everything.

4.16g sugar   36.32g protein
Ingredients (1 portion)
2 chicken meatballs
40g arugula
1tbsp sliced black olives 1/4 avocado
1/2 tomato
1serving caesar dressing

23. Chili Con Carne & Veggies +Egg

442 calories 32.6g fat 18.03g carbs 7.2g fiber   7.32g sugar   22.41g protein
Top 1/3 of the chili with sliced avocado, diced to- mato and sliced hard boiled egg. Enjoy!
Ingredients (1 portion)
1/3 portion chili 1/4 avocado 1slice tomato 1hard boiled egg

CPSIA information can be obtained
at www.ICGtesting.com
Printed in the USA
BVHW011655220221
600779BV00007B/469